Praise for *Path*

"Matthew Sweigart's new book provides a fresh look on a subject too often taught using only boring charts and lists. In *Pathways of Qi*, Matthew takes the reader along on his own personal journey. Although it reads a lot like a novel the text includes an in-depth presentation of the subject. Matthew explains both the scope and the details he has discovered and become familiar with inside the body's electromagnetic field. A very worthwhile read for students, professionals, and even potential clients of Asian Bodywork Therapy (ABT) and acupuncture."

—Cindy Banker, Founding President of the American Shiatsu Association and Director of the A.O.B.T.A.'s Council of Schools and Programs

"*Pathways of Qi* is an empowering manual on Meridian Therapy providing practical ways to heal yourself and others. If you're interested in healing, this book is vital for tapping the source of your life force."

—Michael Reed Gach, author of *Acupressure's Potent Points*

"A gifted Shiatsu and Qi Gong teacher, Matthew Sweigart harmoniously combines his passion for the healing arts with his lifetime experience with the theories of ancient Chinese philosophy. Written in an easy to understand refreshing way, *Pathways of Qi* is a valuable compendium for practitioners and instructors of different traditions."

—Nilsa Eberhart Diaz, owner of Zen Shiatsu Caribbean Institute, San Juan, Puerto Rico

"Matthew Sweigart's clear illustrations and instructions are enhanced by his wisdom stories that bring these teachings to life. The stories and teachings open your eyes to the Qi that is the source of Life, energy and healing. *Pathways of Qi* is a reference tool, a collection of wisdom, and a gift to humanity. Thank you for taking the time to record your wisdom for current and future generations. A masterpiece!"

—Bonnie Jean Miller, MDI, Kellogg School of Management at Northwestern University

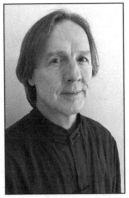

© Tapasya Katarina Stanisaavljevic

About the Author

Matthew Sweigart, AOBTA—CI, (Northern California), is the Director of Education of the American Organization for Bodywork Therapies of Asia. He is also the director and primary instructor of the HeartMind Shiatsu five-hundred-and forty-hour training program offered in Boulder, CO. He began his professional Shiatsu practice in 1988 with the founding of Ohashiatsu Chicago. He currently serves as visiting faculty at Zen Shiatsu Chicago. Matthew is also the author of *Touching Ki, The HeartMind Shiatsu Meridian Gestures* and *Functions Chart, Meridian Qigong,* and several other books and DVDs.

To Write the Author

If you wish to contact the author or would like more information about this book, please write to the author in care of Llewellyn Worldwide, and we will forward your request. Llewellyn Worldwide cannot guarantee that every letter written to the author can be answered, but all will be forwarded. Please write to:

Matthew Sweigart
℅ Llewellyn Worldwide
2143 Wooddale Drive
Woodbury, MN 55125-2989

Please enclose a self-addressed stamped envelope for reply,
or $1.00 to cover costs. If outside the USA, enclose
an international postal reply coupon.

Many of Llewellyn's authors have websites with additional information and resources. For more information, please visit www.llewellyn.com.

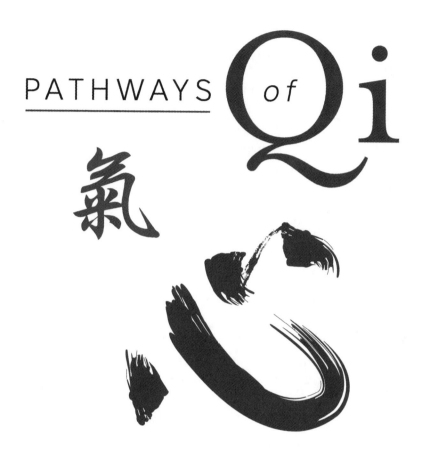

PATHWAYS *of* Qi

Exercises & Meditations to Guide You
Through Your Body's Life Energy Channels

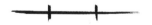

MATTHEW SWEIGART

Llewellyn Publications
Woodbury, Minnesota

First Edition
First Printing, 2016

Book design by Bob Gaul
Cover art by iStockphoto.com/79386175/©Renikca
Cover design by Kevin R. Brown
Editing by Laura Graves

Figure 2 by Llewellyn art department
Figure 15 compilation by Mary Ann Zapalac and Llewellyn art department
All other figures by Mary Ann Zapalac
Interior part page and chapter art by iStockphoto.com/79386175/©Renikca

Llewellyn Publications is a registered trademark of Llewellyn Worldwide Ltd.

Library of Congress Cataloging-in-Publication Data
Names: Sweigart, Matthew, author.
Title: Pathways of Qi : exercises & mediations to guide you through your
    body's life energy channels / Matthew Sweigart.
Description: First Edition. | Woodbury : Llewellyn Worldwide Ltd, 2016. |
    Includes bibliographical references.
Identifiers: LCCN 2016024834 (print) | LCCN 2016030779 (ebook) | ISBN
    9780738748221 | ISBN 9780738750064 ()
Subjects: LCSH: Qi (Chinese philosophy)
Classification: LCC B127.C49 S94 2016 (print) | LCC B127.C49 (ebook) | DDC
    181/.11—dc23
LC record available at https://lccn.loc.gov/2016024834

Llewellyn Publications
A Division of Llewellyn Worldwide Ltd.
2143 Wooddale Drive
Woodbury, MN 55125-2989
www.llewellyn.com

Printed in the United States of America

Contents

Part 2: Working with Meridians through Touch, Meditation, and Qigong

Art List

Introduction

When I was a boy, my physical education began with physical games and activities conducted on the broad lawns of the contiguous backyards of my hometown neighborhood in Dayton, Ohio. My favorite activities were tumbling, somersaults, cartwheels, and all manner of physical feats. My father had been a champion gymnast in his school years, winning the all-around gold medal in his senior year of high school. His natural and trained athletic skill and his joy of living was passed down to all my brothers and sisters and me, and I see it as the early beginnings of my own path into my career as a movement and life energy therapist.

As I grew to be a young man, joyful boyhood games grew into my dedication to an active lifestyle and a fascination with what makes the body work. This found its natural expression for me in music, gymnastics, and dance. I spent many an hour in rehearsal halls and performance stages in secondary school, community theater, college, and into the professional world of stage production. I loved being in my body, singing and dancing and acrobatically moving about. Performance arts gave me an exciting exhilaration and a deep feeling of the life energy flowing through an active body.

My enthusiasm for the performance arts drove me into my early career in the theater, where I worked backstage in theatrical production in my twenties. Now backstage is an exciting and extraordinary kind of place. My natural affinity for a healthy, vital body, mind, and spirit led me to interact with many colleagues in a supportive way. Actors, singers, and dancers use their bodies as their instrument, and as such are always eager to care for it, and refine its capabilities. It was in this light I first learned the arts of assisted stretching and manual therapy practices, what one might consider to be "massage," but something really much more than just a relaxing, luxurious experience.

I was always interested in improving performance and assisting the body in being healthy, vital, and capable of inspirational expression. I found I had a natural talent for promoting natural and optimal energy flow through the body. And with that talent, I found myself helping out the performers with whom I worked. I supported many a singer to relax and perform at their best, dancers to recover from minor injuries so they could stay on their feet, and actors to be grounded and embodied. And the secret to my success I will share with you in these pages was my sensitivity for and work with the meridian pathways of qi as passed down by the traditions and sages of China and Japan.

Interestingly, my first introduction to meridians came through my sister-in-law, Kiki Sweigart. Kiki had a stellar competitive career as a distance runner. The marathon was her specialty event. At the peak of her career, she was ranked in the top ten women runners in the world. I spent a good deal of time running with her in my early adult life. I'll never forget trying to keep up with her as well as following her coaching to bring out my best performance.

It was on one of our runs that she noticed me struggling along and gave me a simple instruction: "You need to open your meridians!" I was intrigued.

As it happens, she didn't elaborate a great deal on what a meridian was or how opening it could help me, but her instruction planted a seed—I became aware of the pathways of life energy, like rivers running through the body. With these rivers' opening could follow a release of exactly the energy one would need to persevere, continue in the face of a challenging performance, and access a deep reserve of support for achieving a goal.

From that small seed has grown this entire work. The meridians are a remarkably powerful and surprisingly accessible personal awareness system. It is my intention to help make these simple, yet profound and sophisticated pathways of qi a part of the regular vocabulary of the body. Just as we are taught fingers, hands, wrists, forearms, elbows, shoulders ... so too do I want us to be able to converse about the body's front, back, and side meridians; the yin and yang flows of life energy; and learn the interconnections of each of our "body parts" as expressions of qi.

I'm happy you are with me on this wonderful journey; I invite you into the beauty and wonder of the body electric and the ways in which qi flows through your body along recognizable channels of flow. When you begin to see these channels and their intricate interconnections, I know that a whole new world of perception will open up for you. I have trained thousands over thirty years, and each time the awareness of the pathways dawns upon a student, they light up with a new enthusiasm for life and its endless possibilities.

In this book I will guide you on a journey through the twelve primary channels. Along the way we will meet and greet the many functions of the body, and discover tools for reading and working with the signs and symptoms of our bodily sensations.

The word *meridian* is a convenient term, but ultimately does not do the pathways justice. It was coined by Western mariners when first arriving in China and learning of the Chinese medical model. In the European year 1027, Chinese medical experts crafted a statue known as the Bronze Man. This bronze figure had traced upon its form the pathways of the energy channels as they flow up and down and across the surface of the body. It reminded the Western mariners of their nautical charts and the meridian lines of latitude and longitude.

The word stuck, and ever afterwards the pathways of qi have been referred to as meridians. Technically, "meridian" is not a very accurate term; the word literally means "an imaginary line on the surface of a body." As you will see, however, the pathways of qi are anything but imaginary. In this work I will demonstrate to you that the points and placement of the channels are actually very deliberate and keen. These channels have a very real life presence, and their location on the body shows up as a powerful correlation and reflection of the very real functions they perform.

So, just as my sister-in-law planted a seed with the simple phrase, "You need to open up your meridians," I hope to plant that seed in you and provide you with the soil, water, and sunlight to grow that seed into a mature working knowledge of the profound and delightful pathways of qi in the human being. Welcome to this journey! Let's get started.

Qi, Meridians, and the Three Treasures

As we begin our journey, we need to place a few key concepts in mind regarding the nature of life energy and how we see and experience it. In three decades of working with these concepts, I have been blessed to be able to study with many great teachers and scholars and interact with a network of professionals who carry on the tradition of teaching these essential energy arts. Of particular power, I learned the powerful practice of *qigong*, literally translated as "energy cultivation." Fundamental to qigong, and to our study here is the understanding of the Three Treasures of life energy: the jing, the qi, and the shen.

Roughly speaking, jing, qi, and shen are equivalent to body, mind, and spirit. Jing is the most physical expression of vital energy, and it shows up as the actual tissues of our body, our size, shape, gender, and ethnicity. And our physical tissues too, like blood vessels, muscles, sinews, and all the working tissues of the body can be described as expressions of jing essence.

Qi is a more immaterial quality of vital energy. As a point of terminology, "qi" is used to name the inherent energy in all things. Its nature can be considered related to thoughts and feelings, experiences we can all agree that we have but are not so tangible that we can grasp and hold on to them in the same way we can touch the physical body.

This expression of qi is correlated here to the idea of mind, the very thoughts, inspirations, and ideas that spring forth from consciousness. In the Chinese language, the word *xin* is the word for "mind" and also "heart." It is not just mind, it is not just heart, it is both! It is what we call "heartmind." Xin represents thoughts and feelings together. This concept of the heartmind is the body/mind connection, central to the material covered in this book. This is the direct realm of qi movement in the human being. Qi can be seen directly expressed as the energy of our thoughts and feelings. And as it flows through our meridian pathways, it directs our vital essence and the expression of who we are and everything we are here to do in this life.

Shen is the spirit, the ethereal essence that resides within through and around all things. Without entering into a theological argument or position, shen can be considered the breath of life itself and the deep mystery of the complex interweaving of all things, the sun, the water, the growing things, and all the living creatures of the earth, the planets, stars, and all the orbiting bodies of the universe, the ever expanding and swirling masterpiece of the universe itself.

It is these three treasures that are at the foundation of this work and the understanding I transmit to you here. Qi is the energy of thoughts and feelings that flows through the pathways. It guides the jing, the tissues of your being, in their full expression of your life and flow. And the shen (your spirit) guides and inspires the flow of qi. This is the vital energy moving through the pathways. This is the work of opening your meridians; the consciousness with which we can open to the flow of life and bring forth the best of all that we can be. To this end, I humbly offer this vision of life energy flowing smoothly and freely through your body, mind, and spirit, your jing, qi, and shen, and all the powerful benefits that can be derived from this vital awakening.

How This Book Is Organized

Pathways of Qi is organized to bring the powerful insights of the meridian and five element system of natural energy into your life. It has long been my wish to make the language of meridians a household understanding. The meridians are extremely powerful and ultimately not difficult to grasp. For many centuries, this knowledge of the meridian channels has been reserved for a professional elite. Here in this work, I offer to help make this wisdom available to everyone with an interest toward self-care and self-understanding.

Of particular note, this availability comes through in the special, clean, clear, and direct affirmations I have crafted for each channel. These affirmations articulate in one or two simple sentences the core action of each meridian channel. By internalizing these affirmations and repeating them in your daily practice you will be supporting the clear and balanced functioning of your meridians.

With these affirmations and the images provided, my goal is to pull the meridian teachings off the shelves of medical academia and into the daily life of the average, intelligent, aware person. I bring you not dry, technical, clinical textbook illustrations but living, moving images of the meridians in motion. In these pages you will see the meridians and their active points depicted in action as well as gestures showing the use and function of each channel simply and accessibly. Also included are day-to-day affirmations in easy to understand language.

In the first section, I will guide you through the regular meridian system channel by channel and show you that moving through the system can be like riding a subway system with twelve different branches or lines, and 365 station stops. Riding the system from beginning to end will lead you on a traverse of the many and varied regions and landscapes of your body. In so doing you will come into an intimate knowing of your body and how it works in relation to your heartmind and daily life.

As a key aspect of the journey, I will illuminate myriad points on your body, and reveal their functions and uses in such a way that you will see how they fit into the overall whole. You will also be shown the amazing common sense and keen insights you can use immediately for optimal performance and awakening of a deep and true knowledge of the various experiences of your life. What I would like by the end of the first section is that you have a strong foundation and the beginnings of a working understanding of your body's pathways of qi.

In the second section of the book, I will help you build that working understanding into a set of practical exercises you can do to take the study out of your head and directly into a felt sense of your pathways of qi in action. In this section you will take a journey through the discernment of excess and deficient energy patterns and how they can affect your overall balance. You'll learn to begin to feel the quality of energy in your meridian pathways and ways to directly affect that energy. Through the practice of brushing, tapping, and palpating, you'll experience what my students call the "qi high": you'll feel giddy and light and more alive than you have ever felt.

I'll then take you on a dive deep into the study of personality using the powerful teachings of six divisions of yin and yang. In this study you will begin to see how your energy truly makes you who you are. You'll inquire deeply within to see if you are more passionate, more sentimental, lustier, or more persnickety. And we will look at these qualities and begin to understand them as a reflection of the qi energy flowing in your pathways.

To sweeten that journey, we'll dive even deeper utilizing guided meditation to take us into a deep felt sense of the five element energy animating all life. Rooted in the deep time-tested understanding of the five elements and how they govern and influence all life as we know it, these meditations will awaken primal energies that help you develop every aspect of your being into the best that you can be.

Finally, I'll get you on your feet and get you moving. With Classical and Meridian Gesture Qigong movements, you will discover a complete system of energy self-care that is time-tested and proven effective to meet and treat any situation that life has sent you. This practical, simple, profound system activates the energy systems in every part of your body, heartmind, and spirit, promoting balance and a heightened self-understanding that is found only in the most profound and insightful practices of the world.

I believe you will find here that the flow of energy from the five elements in nature, through the six divisions of yin and yang, to the twelve regular channels of energy flow in the human being, provides a wonderfully intricate vehicle for understanding the patterns of human life. When we are aware of the patterns, we can see harmony and dissonance. We can learn to emphasize harmony for optimal well-being and bring patterns of dissonance back into balance.

To truly grasp the import of this work will take practice and dedication over time, and an investment of your attention and energy such as you may never have invested before. But I'm here to say that this journey is joyous, and begins to pay dividends from the very first day you put it to use. And with continued practice over time it reveals deeper and deeper, more and more gratifying levels of revelation and insight.

A balanced harmonious nature is our birthright, and modern life can easily pull us out of this natural balance. Sometimes we deliberately take ourselves out of balance, say through intoxication or overindulgence, and then experience the journey back to balance as we sober up or complete the digestion process. Injury or illness also can interrupt and throw us off-balance. Then we seek healing and medicines that assist us in restoring lost equilibrium. The good news is that when trained, our consciousness can grant us the ability to shift and change patterns at will. My offering here is that cultivating your pathways of qi provides a full range of healing interventions that can help you deal with many and varied journeys of dissonance in a safe, natural, holistic, and effective way.

Part 1

The Twelve Regular Meridian Channels

In this first part of our journey, let's get acquainted with the twelve regular meridians. I invite you to approach your body as if it were an organization with a set of very clear departments, each dedicated to the various tasks of your life. I want you to come to know these various departments in a deep and personal way. The twelve regular channels fundamentally describe all the various working systems of being a human being in a living body.

The Life Energy Matrix and Its Functional Layers

As we dive into body of the work, I want to explain the basics in more detail. Qi describes a concept that comes to us from China, synonymous with life energy. This energy permeates all that we are aware of in the cosmos. It is ever present in nature as well as human nature. In the human, this life energy serves to animate and govern all the functions of the human being, from digestion to higher cognition. The ancient Chinese medical system describes a network of energetic pathways or meridians that run throughout the human being, animating all the various functions necessary to the life of the organism.

When we look at these energetic pathways and their material expression, we see an interconnected matrix of the energetic organization of our human form. This book is about exploring that energetic matrix, making sense of it for modern seekers, and displaying some of the benefits that knowledge of the matrix can offer in our pursuit of health, wellness, understanding, and optimal human functioning.

As we approach the topic of studying the matrix of the meridian channel system of Chinese medicine it is important to establish a couple of definitions that will guide us on our journey. First and foremost is the word meridian itself, and the ways in which we understand what a meridian is. And secondly, qi energy, what it is and how we think, feel and experience it. Let's look at the latter first, because it is the "stuff" that flows through the channels of the system, and by knowing what the channel carries, our understanding of the channel itself is clarified.

The concept of qi is deeply rooted in Chinese philosophical history and understanding. It is not within the scope or intention of this work to fully explore all the permutations and expressions of qi. What is most vital to our discussion is to understand qi as an animating, governing force of life. As an animating, governing force, qi is pervasive. It is in evidence wherever and whenever we turn to look, and at the same time it can be unseen and elusive. Qi has many forms and manifestations.

In nature we see qi in all things, from the sustaining still presence within rock and mountain to the rushing torrent of the cataract. Qi shows itself in all natural phenomena of the earth. In the universe qi shows up in all observed phenomena—from the gross movements of the planets around the sun, to the burning of the sun itself, to the quantum levels of atomic particle physics—qi can be seen as the force within it all.

In the human body, as in all animate forms, qi is present as well. It is conceived of as that which animates and governs all the many functions of our being, physically, mentally, and spiritually. From sleeping and waking, digestion and elimination, to higher mental and emotional functioning, qi is the guiding force. When qi is clear and flowing properly, we have health and wellness, when it is blocked from flowing, or has become polluted or distorted, we have dis-ease or anti-wellness.

Now as qi flows through our body it is differentiated into various forms and disseminated throughout the body. As it enters certain pathways known as meridian channels, it becomes known as meridian channel qi. This highly specialized qi flowing through the channels has the task of governing the particular functions of the body, heartmind, and spirit related to the channel in question. The channel system circulates qi throughout the body from deep structures in the internal organs to surface pathways in the muscles, tendons, and cutaneous regions. The channels actually serve to link the deeper aspects of the body to the more superficial aspects.

There are many different kinds of channels within our human being, including regular channels, tendino-muscle channels, connecting vessels, divergent channels, and extraordinary vessels, and all are accessed through some 365 acupoints. In this work we will be studying the twelve regular channels, their trajectories, acupoint locations, and range of functionality. As we study, we will hold the understanding that each meridian channel can be seen as providing governing qi energy to its own range of functions on all levels of the body, heartmind, and spirit. Each channel has its own particular tasks to perform and those distinct tasks are woven into the extraordinary fabric of overall relationship to the whole.

The twelve regular channels have been correlated to the physical organs, and have become known by the name of the viscera most closely related to the range of functions that it governs. These are known in the classical nomenclature as the Zang-Fu. There are ten viscera of note: the Lung, Large Intestine, Stomach, Spleen/Pancreas, Heart, Small Intestine, Bladder, Kidney, Gall Bladder, and Liver. In addition to these ten, two systems identified as the Pericardium and Triple Warmer round out the system of twelve. These latter two have no identified organ correlate but rather define a range of identifiable functions.

Now the channel systems of Chinese medicine indeed have full medical and clinical applications, and a deep study of the systems is the foundation for a serious career as a doctor of Chinese medicine. Yet it is not the intention of this book to train you at the medical level. Rather, my intention is to open you up to the very natural level of accessibility to these systems. And in that opening at the natural level, you will be able to discover a powerful ally in your personal care, as well as something you can share with loved ones. And if you are already a helping professional, you will find this knowledge system a powerful ally in your ability to provide truly outstanding care to your clients and patients.

Because the meridians are named after physical organs, it may be easy to get confused that we are referring simply to physical structures of the body. I assure you this is not the case, and an important point to be clear about. The meridian itself is concerned with the governance of a range of functions from physical and mental to emotional and spiritual. And this makes them highly useful and accessible for any and everyone interested in deepening self-understanding.

In ten of the twelve systems, there is a physical organ that is responsible for the physical range of functioning. In two of the systems, there is not. These last two, by not being correlated to physical organs, help us to see that it is important to make sure that we are not confusing meridians with organs. Organs are physical structures acting on the material level; meridians represent a range of energetic function acting on material, as well as non-material levels.

As we study the meridian channels, we will find that each one follows a particular pathway along the surface of the body that can be related to the range of functions for which it is responsible. And along the pathway, acupoints can be seen as entry and exit points through which the qi within the channel can be accessed and manipulated. A variety of methods from exercise and meditation, to acupuncture and acupressure, to diet and herbs have been developed over the years to make use of the meridians and their acupoints to assess and treat a multitude of conditions of the body, heartmind, and spirit.

This work is an in-depth exploration of the range of functioning for each of the twelve regular channels. Along the way we will be glimpsing how the meridian channels fit into the larger theory of the five element energy transformations and a somewhat deeper look at the six divisions of yin and yang. The theoretical knowledge is presented so as not to limit its application in any way, but rather to provide the foundation understanding necessary for use of the meridian system in a variety of personal self-care and therapeutic settings.

The focus of this work is primarily on the meridian channels and functions. On this journey, it is important to realize that the meridian channels are an expression of natural energies that govern and animate all life on the planet. In Chinese philosophy and cosmology these energies are identified as the five elements: Fire, Earth, Metal, Water, and Wood. In a later chapter, we will engage in an entry-level journey into the five elements and let that take us to a deeper grasp of meridian function.

As we set out, please bear in mind that we are ultimately looking at an interconnected and seamless whole system rather than simply breaking things down into constituent parts. Ultimately body, heartmind, and spirit are one, and all the various functions deeply interwoven. Seeing the system as an interconnected whole helps the development of the insight necessary to perceive patterns of harmony and dissonance as they arise. This is a most important and critical skill. It is not simply that the individual part is singled out for treatment but rather treatment of the individual symptom is seen in the light of its affect on the whole person and on the re-establishment of equilibrium.

Chapter 1

An Overview of the Twelve Regular Meridian Channels

We start the process of opening your meridians by tracing the pathway of qi through the entire twelve meridian sequence with beginning and ending points, following the direction of energy flow and the body's major landmarks. In later sections we'll break it down even further and go through each meridian in greater detail.

The Twelve Regular Channels as One Meridian Flow

In order to see the whole rather than the part alone, it is useful to embrace the concept that there is really only one meridian. Qi energy flows through this one meridian, fulfilling its task of animating all the functions of the body, heartmind, and spirit.

As I describe the way qi essence flows through the body, I want you to begin to see the living expression of your life energy as it is expressed through the various parts of your body and the way in which those various body parts are a direct reflection of the tasks that you perform in life. As the qi of life takes on each of the various tasks of life, we find a fully interconnected holistic pattern of energy flow. In this flow, all the functions have all the energy they need. As we look at these varying functions, we find distinct qualities for each of the twelve regular channels, we see each as distinct "functional units" of energy, yet at the same time, we must always keep our mind open to the deep interrelationships of all the units into one whole flowing system.

Following the traditional trajectories of each energy flow along the surface of the body, from one functional unit to the next in accordance with the daily cycle of energy flow, and seeing how its pathway is a direct reflection of its purpose, we also find that where one meridian ends, the next one begins in close proximity. Like transfer stations in a subway system, connecting vessels between the meridians takes the energy from one channel to the next, making for a seamless flow. As a result, the twelve regular meridian channels link together into one meridian flow.

We'll start with quick, broad brushstrokes, following the meridians in the classical direction along the daily cycle, to lay in the overall pattern of the one meridian flow. As we progress deeper in this work, we will explore the functions of the major body parts through which they flow and correlate these parts to the overall function of each channel. We'll stop at many traditional points, exploring names, meanings, and usage as an illustration of the functional range of the meridian. As the journey unfolds, the multi-layered intelligence of the system reveals itself in profound and beautiful ways.

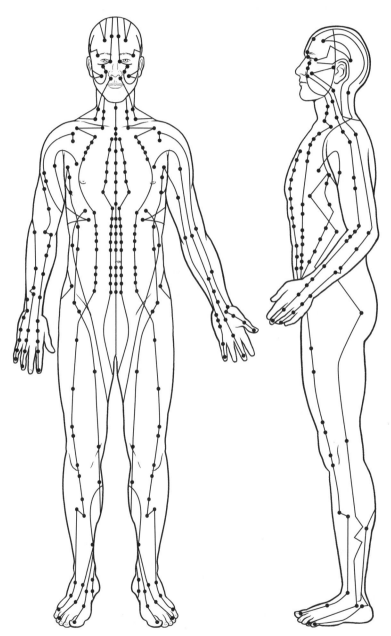

Figure 1: The Twelve Meridians.

Think of the meridian system like a subway map of a modern city. Indeed in ancient China the system of qi channels in the body was conceived during what is now known as the Canal period of Chinese history, that is, a time when a canal system connecting the entire kingdom was created so that goods from one region could be transported to others. This transportation system assured the overall health of the whole kingdom by allowing each to draw from one another's strengths in times of need. So too in the human body can we see that all systems working harmoniously together makes for optimal health. When one system is suffering, another stronger system can assist and support. The meridian system links all the working systems of the body into a coordinated whole.

The coordination of the body's meridians isn't willy-nilly but actually vastly sophisticated. Chinese philosophers observed many natural cycles, among them the natural rise and fall of energies of the day and night that correlated to the body's natural functions. What resulted is what we know today as our internal clock or the circadian rhythm of meridian energy flow.

Thinking of the meridians as a series of one-way subway lines, let's take a journey through the pathways, following the daily clock cycle as they move through the body. As you do this, become acquainted with the beauty, thoroughness, and sophistication of the channel system. Later we will fill in the details of each meridian's range of functions. You'll begin to awaken a deep and brilliant awareness of the way your body and all its systems work together in an intricate harmony.

Channel 1, Lung Line

We start our subway ride through the one meridian flow by jumping on the Lung line, a traditional starting place. The lung is said to be the most evolved of the internal organs, and it is the one whose functioning marks the beginning of our life journey as independent human beings, when we take our first breath. It's a good place to begin.

The Lung line trajectory first manifests on the surface of the body in a point called the Central Treasury, our starting point. It lies on the front, upper torso, just under the clavicle, in the pectoralis major muscle just outside the second rib. From Central Treasury, the Lung line rises up to the clavicle, moves out through the anterior deltoid muscle of the shoulder (the front of the shoulder pads) to the front edge of the biceps, crosses the elbow crease, and runs down along the radius bone where you can see a color change line, from elbow to wrist. It crosses the wrist and runs through the muscle of the thumb to its final point, the Little Merchant, the last point of the Lung line at the base of the thumb nail.

Channel 2, Large Intestine Line

Following the daily cycle flow, the next manifestation of the one meridian is the Large Intestine. And so to continue the flow, we make a transfer from the Lung line over to the Large Intestine line. We hop on the line at its first point, the Yang Merchant, at the base of the nail of the index finger. From there it flows back up the arm along the brachio radialis muscle, crosses the elbow, rises along the upper arm between the bicep and the tricep, and crosses through the deltoid muscle into the shoulder (you can hear the squealing wheels of the Lung line running the opposite direction as the two lines come very close to one another in the shoulder). The Large Intestine line then crosses the front of the neck, passes through the jaw, and finally reaches the end of the line at its last point, Welcome Fragrance, a point just lateral to the nose.

Channel 3, Stomach Line

From there, we transfer to the first point of the Stomach line. We have to walk a little bit between stations from Welcome Fragrance to Tear Receptacle, the first point of the Stomach line just under the eye. From the eye, the Stomach line carries us down the face past the nose and the mouth, loops around through the jaw line (you can hear the mastication, as the teeth do the first job of bringing food into the body), and then rises up to the temple where we notice our mind deciding whether what we have is good food to eat. Having decided in the affirmative, the Stomach line then progresses down again passing through the throat, the breast, traversing the belly, and sweeping out to proceed down the front of the thigh into the leg. It reaches its final destination at Severe Mouth, the nail bed of the second toe.

Channel 4, Spleen/Pancreas Line

From Severe Mouth we hop over to the big toe to pick up the Spleen/ Pancreas line at its first point, Hidden White. Here at the base of the big toe's nail we begin our ride on the Spleen line. This line carries us back up the leg, right along the trough between the shin bone and the calf muscle into the knee joint, continuing up onto the front aspect of the thigh. It crosses over the Stomach line as it moves through the inguinal triangle at the hip and continues to rise up through the abdomen, into the chest, skirts around the breast tissue almost reaching up to the Central Treasury point, but then tails down to its final destination point, the Great Embracement in the side ribs in the sixth intercostal (between the ribs) space on the midaxillary (straight down from the center of the armpit) line.

Channel 5, Heart Line

We've now completed the Spleen line run, so let's transfer over to the Heart line at the point known as Highest Spring to continue our one-meridian flow. From the Highest Spring at the center of the axila (the armpit), the Heart line cuts along the underside of the bicep, passes through the inner elbow, rides along the ulna (the forearm bone on the pinky finger side) to the wrist and hand, reaching its last point, the Lesser Rushing at the base of the pinky finger's nail.

Channel 6, Small Intestine Line

Transferring to the next line in the journey is a simple hop across the nail bed of the pinky finger. We jump from the Lesser Rushing to Lesser March, the first point on the Small Intestine line. Beginning with the pinky finger, this line runs us back up along the ulna to the elbow, crosses into the triceps to ride up to the shoulder, crosses through the shoulder blade, curves over to the top of the back to the spine, rings around the neck to go through the jaw line, enters the face, and finally ends its run at Palace of Hearing, just outside the ear.

Channel 7, Bladder Line

From the Palace of Hearing, we have another small little walk to continue our journey through the one meridian. We need to cross from the ears to the eyes once more, this time to the inner eye and the first point of the Bladder line known as Bright Eyes. From this auspicious starting point at the inner canthus of the eye, we ride the Bladder line up the forehead, over the top of the head, and down the back of the head to the base of the skull. At the base of the skull the line splits into dual channels on each side of the spine, and flows strongly down the back in four lines (two on each side of the spine). The lines pass through many points in the back of the torso and careen on down the back of the thigh to rejoin at the back of the knee. The unified Bladder line then crosses down the calf along the outside of the foot and comes to its final stop at Extreme Yin, at the base of the pinky toe's nail.

Channel 9, Kidney Line

Here at the bottom of the body, we'll now need to make our way back up. In the one meridian flow, our next journey will be on the Kidney line. We take our transfer from Extreme Yin to Bubbling Spring, the first point on the Kidney line, found at the very bottom of the foot.

From there the Kidney line carries us up through the instep, to the inner ankle, up the inner calf, and into the deep inner thigh. From deep in the thigh, it crosses forward to the pubic bone where it carries us on a journey up the front of the abdomen, just a half-inch off the centerline. At the rib cage it widens out to the sides of the sternum, and we make our way to the end of the Kidney line at the Elegant Mansion, nestled in the edge of the sternum above the first rib and just under the collar bone.

So far we've ridden eight of the twelve lines, a full two-thirds of the journey through the one meridian flow. It's nice to take a little rest at the Elegant Mansion before we continue our journey.

Channel 10, Pericardium Line

Take your time, remember to hold on to your transfer, and when you are ready we'll take a little walk from the collar bone down to the breast. There we will find the first point of the next line at the Heavenly Pool, just an inch to the outside of the nipple. We note that this is the Pericardium line. Coming very close to the Lung line, the Pericardium line crosses over the anterior deltoid muscle of the shoulder, traces a course right through the middle of the bicep, through the middle of the forearm, crosses the wrist to the center of the palm, and finally reaches its terminus at the Central Hub in the belly of the flesh at the tip of the middle finger.

Channel 11, Triple Warmer Line

From the Central Hub, we simply skip with our transfer one finger over to the ring finger. Here we hop on the Triple Warmer line at its first point, Rushing Pass. The journey starts up the back of the hand, the backhand stroke of the arm, to the belly of the tricep, to the shoulder where we cross the great trapezius muscle and rise up the side of the neck. From there we travel behind the ear all along the hairline until we reach the temples where we cross over to the final point on the line, the Silk Bamboo Hollow at the end of the eyebrow.

It's been a long journey around the whole body (a total of ten lines behind us), we've almost covered every surface region of the body from front to back to side, and now we only have two lines left to complete our journey through the entire one meridian.

Channel 12, Gall Bladder Line

With barely a half-inch to go, we transfer to the first point on the Gall Bladder line, the Pupil Crevice, just outside the orbital socket of the eye. And we're off, for the ride of our life down the Gall Bladder line.

We now wend a jolly path back to the ear, up into the hair, back around the ear to the base of the skull, coursing back up to the forehead, then switching back over the top of the head again to the base of the skull, and down into the shoulders. From the shoulder, Gall Bladder line drops down into the torso to continue its switchback trajectory.

First it crosses the pectoralis and crosses over the Lung and Pericardium lines to points in the side ribs at the breast line. It then jogs out to the front ribs, just under the breasts in the seventh intercostal space. Next, it switchbacks again to the back and the tip of the twelfth rib, and then it crosses forward again through the waist to the front of the hip. With one more switchback it curves around the hip line to the dimple in the buttocks, and from there the Gall Bladder line's tale of switchbacks settles down, and it runs straight down the side of the thigh along the ileo-tibeal band, crosses the side of the knee and follows the fibula down to the ankle, and makes its way down the top of the foot. It then completes its thrilling trajectory at the final point, Yin Portal of the foot at the base of the nail of the fourth toe.

Channel 12, Liver Line

Taking a deep breath, we're ready for the last run of the one meridian journey. We make our transfer over to the great toe once more where we catch the Liver line at its first point, the Great Pile. From the Great Pile the Liver line carries us back up the body, traversing the top of the foot, up the shin, and back into the middle of the calf to the inner knee and up the inside of the thigh to the groin. Passing very near the Spleen line, it crosses the inguinal triangle veering out toward the tip of the eleventh rib in the side body. It then continues by narrowing toward the middle of the torso once more, running to the sixth intercostal space in the lower rib cage just under the breast in line with the nipples. Here the Liver line completes our entire journey through the one meridian at the final point, the Gate of the Cycle.

The cycle now complete, we can rest once more but only for a moment. From here our one meridian rises again to continue on from the first point on the Lung line. When ready, we transfer our attention over to await the next train out from the Central Treasury, and the flow continues.

The Keys to Unlocking the Pattern

As we look at this continuous flow from one channel to the next we see a fascinating repeated pattern as the one meridian transfers from a yin channel in the arm to a yang channel in the arm, and from a yang channel in the arm to a yang channel of the legs and from there to a yin channel in the legs, and back to the next yin channel in the arm. This pattern repeats three times over to cover all twelve of the regular channels of energy flow. The energy matrix is vast and detailed, and takes time to understand and assimilate. So, please don't worry if you are a little confused right now. We will go over this pattern several times in several ways throughout the course of this book, and in the repetition of the basic pattern you will find your way into the system and make it your own.

Use the charts, do the exercises, find the points on the channels, and awaken a multi-dimensional understanding of the system. Learn to see the points not just in space but also in time. See them as treasure troves of information about the movement of body, heartmind, and spirit throughout a lifetime. When you can see the meridian channels not so much as nouns but as verbs, the system will begin to come alive for you. After all, it is a living system best discovered through your own felt experience. Following is an example of this multi-dimensional approach from my own experience.

I was once hiking in a beautiful tropical wilderness. I wasn't wearing the proper footgear for the terrain; that day, I was wearing rope sandals! If I'd just been hanging around the beach, I would have been fine, but I was in the backcountry hopping from boulder to boulder. Sure enough, one particular boulder had a nice, smooth, inclined face, and my rope sandals turned into mini-sleds. I slid off the boulder to an eight-foot drop and I landed flat footed.

Oh, my ankle screamed at me! (It wasn't both ankles, just my left.) Luckily nothing was broken; I could still hike my way out of that canyon but it was painful as could be. After my return to civilization, I went to a bodywork therapist who applied some brilliant acupressure to a point on my injured ankle. This particular point is on the Gall Bladder meridian. Now, the Gall Bladder meridian as we'll learn below has everything to do with the acts of decision-making, responsibility, reliability, and to a certain extent, flexibility. As the therapist held this point, slowly the many stories of injury to my left ankle came up for review. It was like my ankle tissue was the repository for a cellular-level memory of a whole continuum of accidents and injury. And it became fairly clear fairly soon that each incident had to do with some level of rather poor decision-making on my part.

The healing revealed that it was time for me to finally take some responsibility. As the therapist stayed with the Gall Bladder point and all these memories came up for review, slowly the pain in the ankle began to release. At some point, moisture gushed out of the point like a spontaneous sweating, and then the pain was completely released.

The thing to note here about this healing is that the point was not just simply like a bad part in a machine. Rather it is a living, growing, evolving structure and function that changes, grows, adapts, and heals over time. When you begin to look at each and every point on the body in this way, you open up the capacity to truly come to know the pathways of qi as a powerful reflection of all the multi-faceted aspects of your life and experience.

Let's explore this system in more detail by looking at the terms "yin" and "yang" and their usefulness in describing the nature of phenomena. Through this, we will also be able to see how an understanding of yin and yang helps us understand the manifestation of the various qi pathways and their functions.

Yin and Yang: The Great Ultimate Nature of the Universe

Yin and yang are terms used to describe all the phenomena in the universe we see, feel, and experience, within, through, and all around. In the very earliest usage, yin referred to the shady side of the hill and yang to the sunny side. From this perspective, you can see that yin and yang are inseparable and co-create one another. We only need open our eyes and ears and feeling senses to awaken the personal experience of yin and yang in life. Yin and yang are the equal, complementary, relative, polar opposite forces of the universe. Together they make the whole.

In a basic body sense, think of internal and external aspects of your being. The internal we see as yin, the external as yang. Take a look at movement and stillness. We see yin as stillness and yang as movement. Extend that to active and inactive. A dormant volcano is yin, an active volcano is yang. Yang and yin complement one another and one does not exist without the other. "Yin" and "yang" are terms used to describe various observed and experienced phenomena and the nature of interconnection. Sleep is less active and therefore yin, and it is coupled with the nighttime. Wakefulness is more active and therefore yang, and correlates to daytime.

Now it is true also that in their co-creativeness, yin and yang are also infinitely divisible. We may say that night is generally yin, but within the night are the nocturnal creatures that become active. We would call this yang within yin. And so too, even in the daylight one may lie down and take a nap, and we would call this yin within yang. And in these examples I invite you to begin to open yourself to the idea that yin and yang are not absolute but exist upon a gradient that moves through time.

The day begins before the dawn with the breaking of the light in the east, and this movement progresses through to sunrise. Still the day is just dawning and then growing until it reaches high noon, and the shadows are at their smallest. Then as high noon passes, and the shadows lengthen, day is waning, and night is beginning. And so night begins with the long shadows of dusk, the setting of the sun, the lingering light deepening slowly into full darkness. And at the fullness of the moonless night, the stars shine out brightly until the sun approaching from the east once more calls forth the dawning of the new day.

The yang of day begins small, grows and grows to its fullness, and then wanes after its peak. The yin of the night also creeps up through the lengthening shadows, grows to its fullness in the deep darkness of the middle of the night, and then gives way once more to the yang rising of the new day. This whole cycle repeats and repeats and repeats in the roundness of life's continuing flow.

You also see these gradual changes in the seasons of the year: the yang of summer gives way through autumn to the yin of winter, which gives way through spring to the yang of summer once more. And even in the winter we can have a summery day, (yang within yin) and in summer a wintry day (yin within yang).

We can also see this gradient in hunger and fulfillment cycles in our human life cycles. When we are hungry, we begin to eat, but the first bite does not satisfy. We continue to eat until we begin to feel satisfied, and then we eat until we are completely satiated. But as we leave the table, within a short while we may already be a little bit hungry, but we wait until we get a little bit hungrier still, until finally we are hungry enough to get food to eat again.

Emerging from these observations you see the yin-yang principle describing the three-part nature of flow: beginning, middle, and end; elder, middle, and youngest; child, adult, elder. Classical Chinese philosophy describes three aspects of yin and yang. For yin they are *Tai Yin*, *Jue Yin*, and *Shao Yin*—the greater, middle, and lesser yin. And for yang, the three aspects are *Tai Yang*, *Shao Yang*, and *Yang Ming*—the greater, lesser, and sunlight yang. Together these are known as the six divisions. They are the gradients of yin and yang, reflecting the way in which things change and move through time and space. These six divisions can be observed in many aspects of life. As we study the pathways of qi, they will show up for us here in the yin and yang gradients of the meridian channels in the front, back, and side meridian lines of the one meridian.

Yin and yang are continually chasing one another's tail, following the endless principle of the way things change through time and space. Yin naturally becomes yang, and yang naturally becomes yin. As yin grows, yang diminishes, and vice versa. The channels of energy flowing through the body governing the various functions of our being are of both yin and yang qualities.

Within the twelve regular channels are six yin channels and six yang channels. The yin energies are more internal and relate to the internal functioning of our solid *fu* organs: the Heart, Spleen, Lung, Kidney, and Liver channels.

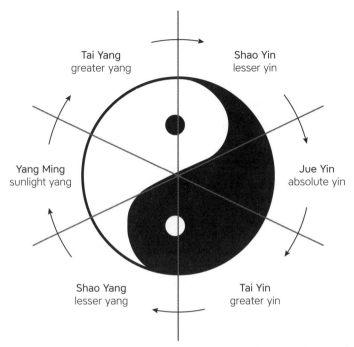

Figure 2: Here we can see the famous symbol of yin
and yang is actually a flow chart depicting the movement
of yin and yang energy transformations over time.

The yang energies are more external and relate to the functioning of our hollow *zang* bowels: the Small Intestine, Stomach, Large Intestine, Bladder, and Gall Bladder channels. These organ networks are further differentiated into the six divisions to distinguish from more superficial to deeper functions. For instance, the Lung and Heart channels are both considered yin but it is apparent that the Lung channel is much more at the surface of our bodies, interfacing directly with the air that surrounds us. The Heart channel lies deeper in the body, at our core, well protected from direct outside influence. So too, does a respiratory condition like the common cold seem more superficially distressful when compared to a condition of the circulatory system such as hardening of the arteries, or arterial plaque.

Remember in this discussion that there are only ten actual physical organs mentioned but twelve differentiated meridian functions. The missing pair of functions is worth special consideration on their own, and they represents one of the great gifts of Chinese medicine to the understanding of human functioning. They are the Pericardium and Triple Warmer channels. These two channels have no physical organ correlation (though the pericardium is often related to the muscle that surrounds the heart). We will explore the functions of this pair of channels in more detail later, but for now it is important to use them to make a distinction between meridians and organs.

A Meridian Is Not an Organ

A meridian in many ways is a nonmaterial energetic quality that has the task of animating and governing various functions in human life. For channels that do have a physical organ correlation, it is important to see that the organ was created in order to fulfill that function at the physical level. For example, consider Stomach: the stomach organ itself is responsible for breaking down food such that it is possible for the body to extract nutrients for biological functioning. But the Stomach channel is much more widely responsible for providing nourishment to the body, heartmind, and spirit overall. Beyond mastication and digestion of food, it is in fact in charge of the entire set of functions—acquisition, preparation, and delivery—of life sustaining product for the body. For that function to be fulfilled, many more aspects of the human form and function such as food crop cultivation, hunting, gathering, cooking, mastication, and swallowing, all are used to support the actual organ in the belly. These are all functions of the Stomach channel. Beyond physical food, consider also appetites we have for spiritual fulfillment, emotional support, intellectual stimulation, and sexual desire. All of these appetites are governed and animated by the Stomach channel.

The Pericardium and Triple Warmer channels also serve their own wide range of functioning in the human form, but what they have to do simply does not correspond to actual, physical organs. The range of functions they serve are primarily in the realm of protection for the body and overall regulation of all the systems including the immune system, blood flow, organ interactions, and the emotional and intellectual matters of interpersonal communication. As we study we might wonder: if there was no correlative physical organ, how did the Chinese know these functions even existed in the body? In the answer to this question we come to appreciate that Chinese medicine is not so much a medicine of form as it is of function. As a culture, they were not anatomists—indeed there were serious restrictions on cadaver dissection. (When we see the ancient drawings of the internal organs, we are often amused at the fanciful figures drawn to represent the organs. Yet many of the drawings are remarkably accurate.) The point is this: Chinese medicine is much more concerned with function rather than physical form. And to guide their understanding of function, Chinese physicians applied their understanding of yin and yang.

As we look at the nature of the six divisions of yin and yang in relation to the channels, we find ourselves looking at the body and three relative corresponding regions of the "front," "back," and "sides." The front is clearly visible when we look at someone face-on, the sides when they turn sideways to us in a striding position and we view both the lateral and medial aspects of their limbs, and the back clearly when we look at them from behind. Though there are some variations on the actual locations of the channels relative to these general bodily regions, the channels and their yin/yang designations generally correspond to the areas of front, back, and side.

The Tai Yin (greater yin) (Spleen and Lung) and Yang Ming (sunlight yang) (Large Intestine and Stomach) energies can be seen easily when looking at the head on approach or "front" portion of the body.

The Jue Yin (absolute yin) and Shao Yang (lesser yang)—related to the Liver and Pericardium, and Triple Warmer and Gall Bladder, respectively—lie in the lateral and medial or "side" aspects of the body. And the Shao Yin (lesser yin) and Tai Yang (greater yang)—related to the Kidney and Heart, and Small Intestine and Bladder respectively—can generally be seen from the "back" view of the body. The upper aspect of the Kidney meridian, with its many points on the abdomen and chest, is the clearest exception to this mapping designation, but even so we draw from the Kidney channel's location in the feet and legs and the kidney organs' position deep in the posterior anatomy of the body that Kidney is indeed a channel of the "back" body.

As we have traveled through the one meridian and seen the way in which the energies of the various channels flow through the body, we may be wondering why they flow in the direction that they flow. The answer to this lies in the classical understanding of yin and yang flow.

Yin energies are the energies of the earth and are said to rise up from the earth into the body. Yang energies conversely are the energies of the heavens or cosmos, and are said to descend from above and course down through the body. To bring that understanding into the flow of channel energy in the body, we need to understand that in the Chinese anatomical position, the arms are extended up over the head. The yin leg channels begin at the feet and rise up into the torso, and the yin arm channels begin in the torso and end in the hands. The yang arm channels begin in the hands and flow into the head and face, and the yang leg channels begin in the face and travel down the body to the feet.

So now we can see that the yin arm channels begin in the torso and flow to the hands. There they connect naturally to the yang arm channels that begin in the hands and flow to the face. There in the face, the yang arm channels connect to yang leg channels that begin in the face and run down to the feet. And in the feet the yang leg channels connect to yin leg channels that begin in the feet and then travel back up the body to end in the torso, where they naturally connect to the yin arm channels once more.

This endless cycle from yin to yang to yang to yin, from arms to legs to legs to arms carries on, day in day out throughout the life cycle of the human being. With an understanding of this natural flow of energy we can begin to watch for signs of the natural flow being disrupted, identify the disruption, and restore the natural flow.

As we have explored the meridians in the order of this daily cycle, we have seen that where one meridian ends, the next one begins in near proximity, supporting the image of one continuous flow of life energy throughout the body. Applying the understanding of the six divisions of yin and yang to the twelve meridians, we discover this revealing pattern in the way the pathway flows from one aspect to the next.

Looking at these six divisions of yin and yang and how they appear in the meridian channels of the arms and legs and the areas of "front," "middle," and "back," we discover the fascinating correlation between the functions they govern and the body parts through which they course. In doing so, we see amazing relationships between body surface and internal functions.

The "front" meridians naturally reflect things about us that are up front, the "back" meridians give us access to deeper aspects of self, and the "side" meridians relate to our flexibility and ability to move from side to side. The front meridians govern our boundaries and appetite, the back meridians relate to our self-awareness and deepest innermost feelings about life and death, and the side meridians govern our self-protection and decision-making faculties. The meridians flow through the body, one leading to the next in a continuous energy circuit, day in and day out for our entire lifetime. This one circuit of the twelve channels makes for one complete traverse of the yin and yang aspects of front, back, and side regions of the body, correlating deeply to the front, back, and side aspects of our entire life.

The Three Layers of Health

Thus the twelve regular channels give us a thorough mapping of the body's subcutaneous energetic matrix and cover a vast range of the human functions. It is important to understand that the regular channels constitute only one major part of the whole system that the ancient Chinese pieced together to describe all the functions of life. To be clear, the regular channels do not cover the entire range of human functions. There are indeed other channel systems that together with the regular channels fully describe the many intricacies of human functioning. In Chinese medicine we additionally study twelve tendinomuscular channels, forty-eight connecting vessels, twelve divergent channels, and eight extraordinary vessels. In this book, our focus is on the twelve regular channels. Details of the other systems are simply beyond the scope of this work but bear mentioning so that you can see the full context in which the regular channels exist. A thorough working knowledge of all these functioning systems gives a deep and complete understanding of the entire range of human functioning, but because all the systems are interrelated and overlap, working with the regular channels alone can provide you with a most powerful tool for accessing all parts of your human experience.

To best understand the place of the twelve regular channels in the overall functioning systems of the human being, let's look to the classical Chinese medical model of three layers of health. Seeing the three-part nature of things is a very powerful tool for understanding how things move and change over time and through space. Just as there are three layers of yin and three layers of yang, there are also these three layers of health. These three layers are known as the reflexive, the conditioned, and the constitutional.

The Reflexive Layer

The reflexive layer of health relates to our innate ability to respond to situations in which we find ourselves in an appropriate way. When we encounter something hot, we pull away. When we hear a loud and threatening noise, we jump. The tendinomuscle channels govern the reflexive layer of health. One could say that this is the most superficial of the three layers, but that is not to diminish its extreme importance. If your reflexes are compromised, it can put you in a very serious situation indeed.

The Conditioned Layer

The conditioned layer of health encompasses the entire range of our learned behaviors; the ways we were taught to behave in the various social and interpersonal situations in which we find ourselves. This layer is governed by the functioning of the twelve regular channels. You could say that this conditioned layer of health is deeper than the reflexive layer.

The Constitutional Layer

Finally, the third layer of health is the constitutional layer. In this layer we are looking at the range of functioning governed by our genetic and karmic endowment or predisposition. In short, it describes the inherent gifts we were born with and what are we meant to be doing in this lifetime with what we have been given. The eight extraordinary vessels govern this layer of health. And here it is easy to see that this might be considered the deepest of the layers of health.

With these three layers of health and the three channel systems correlating to them, we find powerful tools for understanding what is out of balance and how to best go about treating it.

As for connecting vessels, in many ways these can be seen functioning on all three levels, and the divergent channels offer a direct link between reflexive and constitutional layers, giving us the ability to respond in an instant from a deeply innate place. Ultimately all the systems overlap and interconnect, so in working with any one system the power of the whole is accessed as well.

Through this brief overview of the three layers of health, I hope I have given you a good idea of the power and usefulness of a working knowledge of the twelve regular channels of energy flow and how they fit into the picture of overall health. The conditioned layer of health and its many manifestations comprise the majority of our exploration here. So roll up your sleeves and get ready to ride deeper along our journey to help balance and harmonize the life conditions in which you have found yourself.

Developing yourself through balancing the flow of qi through the pathways can help you effectively triumph over adverse conditions and celebrate the arrival of advantageous conditions for all your life experiences. May this knowledge and wisdom help you flourish in all levels of your life experience, penetrating even the most difficult of issues and finding resolution and harmony for your greater happiness, wholeness, and well-being.

Chapter 2

Establishing and Maintaining Boundaries and Exchange

In this chapter we explore the Lung and Large Intestine channels and their function in body, heartmind, and spirit. Note that these lines constitute Tai Yin and Yang Ming as aspects of the Metal elemental force, located in the arms on the front of the body.

Lung Meridian

Hand Tai Yin

The original name for this channel of energy, "Hand Tai Yin" describes the nature of the energy of this channel and where it lies on the body. This is the greater yin energy as it expresses out through the hands, particularly as it flows from the upper torso, down the arm, and out through the thumb. The Lung channel is the Hand Tai Yin organ network of the body.

Metal

Metal is the term given to the elemental quality of exchange and connectivity. It is also attributed to whatever is considered treasure. The Lung organ network is in charge of the inflow and outflow of treasured substances. On a basic level, it is the very air we breathe. Metaphorically, it relates to life's gains and losses through our interrelationship with the environment around us. Metal interconnects our world.

3 to 5 am

There are twenty-four hours in a day and twelve meridians. The ancients discovered that each meridian channel had a peak time that correlated the energy of the time of day with the energy flowing in the channel. The hours of 3 to 5 am are considered the beginning of the energetic day. The Lung organ network is correlated to the beginning of our energetic life with the first breath at birth.

Key Functions

Intake of qi, gaseous exchange with environment

Affirmation

I breathe in the pure qi of the universe, nourishing every cell of my being.

The Lung channel of Hand Tai Yin is the yin aspect of the Metal element in the body, and it runs a course from the torso to the hands. The Lungs govern respiration, the primary fundamental rhythm of life's in-breath and out-breath. As such we can consider it a vessel of exchange with the environment, especially on the gaseous level. On the simplest level, oxygen is taken in and carbon dioxide is eliminated through the lungs. Beyond the internal organ system associated with air exchange, the Lung channel also includes the skin. Considered the largest single organ in the body, the skin represents the borders or boundaries of our physical body. Like the internal lung organs, the skin also breathes the air around us through our many pores. If all our pores were to be sealed off, we would die of asphyxiation.

Taking these basic functions as metaphors for intake and elimination on all levels, we see the Lung channel's sphere of functional influence expanded to include any income or outflow in our lives on all levels—physical, mental, emotional, and spiritual.

With its function and metaphorical understanding in consideration, grasp the image of the Lungs as the manifestation of personal borders. These borders both set us apart from and connect us to the world around us. Let's spell out in some detail the functions governed and animated by the Lung channel of life energy.

Key Characteristics of Functional Range of the Lung Channel

PHYSICAL

The physical range of functions for the Lung channel all relate to the respiratory organ system and functions; breathing in oxygen and breathing out carbon dioxide is its most direct life sustaining function. The scientists who lived in Biosphere II learned very well that the carbon they breathed out, became the food they would eat, and the plants that lived in the Biosphere needed to produce enough oxygen in return for them to be able to survive.[1] This balance is taken for granted in the greater experience of the climate zones and life across the surface of the earth. But in Biosphere II, a sealed enclosure, it became immediately clear how delicate and necessary it is that this be a balanced exchange. So, inhalation, exhalation, bringing the necessary in and letting the necessary out, is a key physical function of Lung channel energy.

---

1   Kara Rogers, Two Years Under Glass: The First Biosphere 2 Mission. *Encyclopedia Britannica Blog*, September 26, 2011.

Beyond this respiratory system, the Lung channel also has physical expression in the skin. The skin has actually been proven to be the largest organ in the body. Skin tissue, lung tissue, and the gut's lining tissue are all made of the same "stuff," epithelial tissue. This marvelous tissue interfaces between internal and external environments, serving as a "boundary" layer. You might think of it like the borders of a country: at the border, the vital work of commerce and exchange takes place. So the skin becomes somewhat of a customs agent for the body. It is semi-permeable in nature. It lets some things in and some things it keeps out. If you sit in a bathtub you won't become bloated with water, but you will absorb minerals from the bath. The skin allows the minerals through, but keeps the water out.

The semi-permeable quality possesses a protective quality by extension. The Chinese call this *wei qi* ("protective qi") and the Lung channel governs its management. It is the first line of defense against pathogenic influences from the outside world. Healthy functioning of wei qi does indeed keep us healthy in our many common interactions with the world around us.

On the last physical layer of Lung channel governance, we now examine the nasal cavity. The sinuses are entry-level access to the lungs, and we can see in their proper functioning that initial "scrubbing" of the air upon intake. The wei qi here in the sinuses is hard at work. If you've ever suffered a sinus infection, you're acutely aware of what can sometimes be a battle zone between the body and the external world. An important fluid in that battle zone is mucous. Indeed mucous is the bodily fluid governed by Metal to include both the Lung channel and Large Intestine functions. With healthy mucous, wei qi is strong. Look for Lung channel in action any time your mucous membranes are inflamed or challenged.

PSYCHOLOGICAL, EMOTIONAL

As we enter into the psychological and emotional realms of life energy as governed and expressed through the qi channel system, we find ourselves simply in the process of using the physical layers as metaphor for these more ethereal functions. The classical Chinese system correlates the organ networks with emotions, and for the Lung channel we find the emotions of grief and sorrow. Take a moment to take a deep breath and consider your own experience of sorrow. You will notice perhaps quite quickly how strong an effect the feeling of sorrow has on your breathing. Choking, sighing, sobbing, crying, and producing copious amounts of mucous while in abject grief all correlate with one another.

You'll note that grief is rooted in loss. Loss is a function of exchange with our environment. Someone or something that was once an integral part of the environment we live and breath in has been taken away, and we are left with a hole in our lining, if you will. The place we had come to rely on, lean on, or press up against is no longer there. Sorrow is the result. Our wei qi needs to be reorganized. Our borders, boundaries, sense of a separate and sovereign self, as well as our connection to all that is comes into question.

Here we enter the rich and profound realm of the psychological and emotional layers of the Lung channel function. As an example, a particularly poignant story arose in one of my classes. My students are all given an assignment early on called "Meridians in Daily Life."

I will encourage you to undertake this assignment for yourself as this journey proceeds. In the assignment, the task is to take one experience from your life that involved some injury to your body and correlate how the injury happened along a given meridian channel as well as the experience you were going through at the time directly correlating to that meridian function.

In the case of the Lung meridian, I recall a direct experience of my own when I had just heard the news that one of my first inspirational teachers had passed away. I was in what I would call a mild level of mourning over the loss. At the time, I was fortunate to be able to receive a shiatsu treatment from a colleague.

As I was receiving the treatment, the practitioner came to the point Lung 6, Maximum Opening, on my forearm. The pressure was exquisite and began to open me up to deeper feelings of grief. I kept asking for more and more pressure on the point.

The practitioner was surprised but agreed. As the pressure sustained and deepened, it took me deeper and deeper into a full experience of the profound loss I was feeling.

SPIRITUAL

We are now brought to the spiritual level of meridian function. At the spiritual level, the Lung channel is concerned with oneness, our connection to all that is, the maintenance of personal space in the midst of the vastness of all space in which we find ourselves, and ultimately the "rightness" or "suchness" of things.

So many times, loss and gain are simply mysterious functions of the universe. The best-laid plans oft go awry, and in such times we are left to surrender into what is so, just as it is no matter what.

This is the Lung channel's high spiritual function. If you find yourself caught in a dilemma between what is so and what you wish were so, your Lung channel may be crying out for attention.

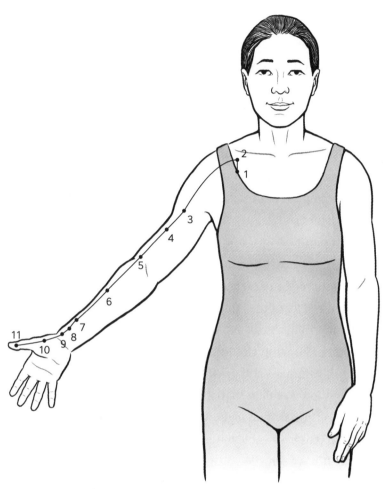

Figure 3: Lung Meridian—Hand Tai Yin.

1. Central Treasury
2. Cloud Gate
3. Palace of Heaven
4. Reaching White
5. Cubit Marsh
6. Maximum Opening
7. Broken Sequence
8. Channel Gutter
9. Great Abyss
10. Fish Belly
11. Little Merchant

The Lung Channel Trajectory

The Lung meridian begins at a point one inch below the collarbone (clavicle), just lateral to the second rib. From here it runs up to the clavicle and crosses laterally to the anterior deltoid. It proceeds down the bicep, into the forearm along the radius, and ends in the thumb.

To feel the entire flow of this meridian in one gesture, start with your hands at your sides, and turn them out. Leading with your thumbs, stretch your arms back, opening your chest and looking up with your head. Take a deep breath and fill your lungs with air while stretching the thumbs back and out.

The first point on the Lung meridian, Lung 1, is known by the name of Central Treasury, as we learned earlier, but it also has the alternate name Center of Gathering, a name that along with its significance reveals a deep insight into the place of the Lung in human life. While holding Lung 1 and rotating your arm in a great arc, you will notice that this is the centerpoint of the rotation. Looking closely at this action, it is important to understand that only humans and primates have the ability to move their arms in this way. It is this ability that allows us to gather things. We gather up our young and run from danger. We gather the grain and the foodstuffs. We gather all that is valuable to us, and sometimes even that which it not so valuable. It has been shown that the first invention of civilization was the vessel, or urn, a place to store whatever we have gathered. We gather things, and because we can do so, we can settle down and stay in one place. This is a major feature of civilization that has put us in a unique place among all the species of the earth.

When we look more literally at the physical aspect of the Lung meridian function, the lungs can be considered gatherers of the air we breathe, bringing it into our body/heartmind/spirit for life support. This point is therefore most auspicious; from here we begin our journey of exploring the human form. In the name, Central Treasury, we also see the connected activity of gathering and dispersing our treasure in our income and expenses. Here, too, is a reflection of the lungs' functions: inhalation and exhalation, intake and expenditure.

From Lung 1, the channel travels upward one inch to Lung 2, Cloud Gate, just inferior to the clavicle. (The anatomical term "inferior" is used as a point of reference to describe a location that is in the direction of downward or "toward the earth" from the referenced landmark, when the body is standing upright.) One of the major functions of Lung energy is to disperse moisture downward through the body. A long, slow, deep breath epitomizes this sense of downward energy flow the Lung governs. With such a breath we slow down and drop inward. The Cloud Gate opens and down comes the rain. Falling rain is often associated with down and introspective times, and it serves as an appropriate representation of the Lung's emotional connection to grief.

From Cloud Gate, the Lung meridian turns out and crosses over the anterior deltoid ("anterior" refers to any thing that is in front; the deltoid is the superficial muscle of the shoulder, the one that shoulder pads accentuate) into the arm where it travels down to the thumb. On its way it passes along the lateral (toward the outside) edge of the bicep in a perceptible trough just anterior to the humerus (the upper arm bone). The bicep allows us to pull and hold things and also release and let things go, a function to which the Lung can be related, as we pull in the in-breath and let go of the out-breath. The first of two points along the bicep is Lung 3, Palace of Heaven. The name evokes images of the vital function of the lungs in gathering nourishment from the air around us. The point is also at the level of the breast, the storehouse of mother's milk that can be used in the treatment of lactation disorders. We see here a relationship between the Lung function of energy intake of air and the intake of food for nourishment. The second point along the bicep is Lung 4, Reaching White. This name is a reference to the Lung meridian's protective function and its place as the first line of contact with the world around us. The color in the name is also related to the Lung meridian. White evokes images of cleanliness, and the lungs best nourish the body with fresh, clean air.

At the elbow crease we find Lung 5, Cubit Marsh or In the Groove. This point can be seen in the action of snapping fingers. The rhythm of the breath is a most fundamental rhythm of human life. Snapping your fingers in a rhythm gets your breath moving in a rhythmic way as well, replenishing your lungs with fresh and pure qi with each breath.

In the forearm, the Lung channel runs from the elbow to the wrist along the edge where the fairer skin of the anterior surface meets the darker skin of the posterior surface. Often, this is also the hairline or freckle line, clearly marking a place of transition from one aspect of our body to another. The darker skin side of this line is associated with the yang or exterior aspects of our being and the fairer skin side with the yin. The Lung is a yin meridian and as such rides right along the edge of the yin aspect of the arm. Along this line we find Lung 6, Maximum Opening, whose name alludes to the Lung's function of being an opening for the coming and going of life. Next we arrive at Lung 7, Broken Sequence, a reference to this point's location, which is slightly deviated from the rest of the line. Interestingly, it is said that energy bursts forth at this point and leaps over to Large Intestine 4, on the next meridian after Lung, thus breaking the flow before the Lung meridian has runs its course.

The meridian resumes its course with Lung 8, Channel Gutter, lying along a stretch of fiber that resembles a narrow passage way. It has depth but is narrow, and therefore is used to treat challenges to the esophagus or windpipe. The name calls to mind the image of moving water effectively from one place to another. This narrow passageway through the wrist is analogous to the relatively narrow transporting passageway of the neck, and it highlights the Lung meridian's job of transporting energy to the meridian system. The Japanese reflect this analogy in their language as well. The Japanese word *kubi* is the word for neck, and *tekubi*, which literally translates as "hand-neck," is the word for wrist. From this analogy, we can see how points of the wrist may all be used to treat conditions of the neck.

At the point where the wrist meets the hand we find Lung 9, Great Abyss, resting in the hollow distal to the head of the radius, the thumb side bone of the forearm (*distal* means "further away from the center of the body"), and proximal to the carpal bones of the wrist (*proximal* means "closer to the center of the body"). This point is used to treat challenges to the thoracic cavity. Rather than a narrow passageway, it is more cavernous, thus the name. Its alternate name, Great Stagnation, speaks to how such pools can become clogged, and indeed this place is likely to experience an excess of stagnant energy. Simply call to mind the feelings in your chest when you have a chest cold or after you have received the heavy news of some great loss in your life, and you can see the range of usages for this point. Also of note is its relation to grip. In times of loss or respiratory distress, there can be an accompanying feeling of weakness.

The Lung meridian continues, crossing the wrist crease on its way into the thumb. If you make a hitchhiking gesture with the arm extended to the back, you get a sense for the overall pathway of Lung energy extending out from the upper chest down the arm to the thumb. And right in the middle of the belly of the thumb muscle is Lung 10, Fish Belly. Here we again observe the phenomenon of a color change line on the skin. The Lung channel rides along this border between the dark and the light, the yang and the yin aspects of the body's exterior. This skin is stretched in the hitchhiking gesture. It is a gesture of a request for a ride, a connection with another human to gift you a lift and take you from one place to another.

It is characteristic of this gesture that the thumb is used and not the index finger. Indeed, the index finger is used to hail a taxi cab, a gesture that signifies the hiring of a driver to render a service for pay. As we will see as we move along into the next meridian, the Large Intestine, these two gestures are a perfect example of the yin and yang aspects of this life function. The hitchhike gesture with the thumb is yin, a request for assistance. The gesture for hailing a cab is yang, an order for service from a paid provider. In both cases we are getting a ride from one place to another, a task within the realm of influence of the Lung and its partner the Large Intestine having the obligation to connect us with our environment.

One final point remains on the Lung channel before we make our journey over to the Large Intestine. Resting at the base of the thumbnail is Lung 11, Little Merchant. This point just oozes with significance related to how we deal with our treasure. Its full significance is evident in relation to Large Intestine 1, Yang Merchant, found at the base of the nail of the index finger. The gesture of rubbing the index finger and thumb together is used to indicate a wish for pay or that something is quite expensive. And of course the opposing thumb and forefinger is a hallmark of the human form, giving us the ability of fine motor movements and attention to detail. It is also another aspect of the Lung and Large Intestine function, to be concerned with the details.

Large Intestine Meridian
Hand Yang Ming
The original name for the channel, Hand Yang Ming describes the energy of Sunlight Yang as it expresses in the front surface of the human form, specifically related to this energetic quality as it flows from the index finger to the nose. The Large Intestine energy is the physical expression of the Hand Yang Ming energy in the organ system.

Metal Element
As with Lung, Large Intestine is also related to the Metal element. It is the element of borders and boundaries, interconnections with our environment, and things of great value. Whereas the Lung is an expression of the yin aspect of Metal, the Large Intestine is an expression of its yang aspect.

The main product of the Large Intestine function is generally regarded as the body's solid waste, but it is also a valuable product for reproducing nutrients in soil.

5 to 7 am

This time of day is granted to Large Intestine energies; many will attest to this being the time of day when a bowel movement is expected and appreciated.

Key Functions

Elimination of stagnation of qi, material exchange with environment

Affirmation

I eliminate that which is no longer of use to me.

The Large Intestine channel of Hand Yang Ming is the yang channel of the Metal element and traces a trajectory from the hand to the face. It is named after the main organ in the body responsible for the elimination of solid waste. It is also the system responsible for water reclamation and the recycling of a few key nutrients such as good cholesterol. Taking this as metaphor, we can develop an understanding of the Large Intestine channel's function on all levels of our being. Like it's yin partner the Lung channel, the Large Intestine governs our boundaries and borders. It is particularly involved in the purging of that which is no longer of use. When it is healthy we see an easy, regular elimination of solid waste; when it is in distress we see signs of constipation or diarrhea. This property can manifest not just physically but mentally, emotionally, and spiritually as well. Letting go and allowing things to pass is a major part of the Large Intestine's functional range. When waste or whatever is in our life that is no longer useful is not being easily eliminated, it is a sign of imbalance in the Large Intestine function. Below we explore many of the basic functions related to the Large Intestine channel.

Key Characteristics of Functional Range of the Large Intestine Channel

PHYSICAL

The obvious physical function of the Large Intestine meridian is the elimination of solid waste from the body on a regular and timely basis. In addition to the elimination of the solid waste, it's important to note the as solid stool is forming in the Large Intestine, the Large Intestine is performing the important role reclaiming water from the digested material. In the absence of this healthy water reclamation we experience the watery stools of diarrhea. And if that continues for too long, we can experience dehydration.

Taking these two functions together, the elimination of solid waste and the intake of digestive water into the system, we can easily understand the organ's relationship to the Lung channel. The inflow and outflow essential to life as conducted by these two channels is their primary physical function in the human being.

PSYCHOLOGICAL, EMOTIONAL

Considering this physical action as metaphor, let's sketch a picture of the psychological and emotional functions of the Large Intestine channel as well. In doing so, we'll find the myriad psychological and emotional reactions that contribute to monitoring ones' environment. Consider the codes, covenants, and restrictions of any gated community or system of governance (to include law and order), and we observe an effort to keep things in order or watch over how affairs are conducted.

We get a sense of stability through the predictability of everyone in an environment following an agreed upon set of rules, standards, ethics, and moral considerations. This is the healthy realm of Large Intestine function in society.

And just like the Lung, the Large Intestine also has its part in grief. Consider the kind of grieving "constipation" or "paralysis" that can set in: the inability to move forward (or at all) due to the heavy and debilitating feeling of loss. Letting go of a major loss makes us feel as though some heavy hand forces the loss upon us, such as in the tragic or sudden death of a child. Experiences like these present themselves as manifestations of energies related to the Large Intestine channel, manifesting in the body as stiffness and lower back aches, pains that lay us low with grief's heavy burden.

Lighter perhaps than such heavy grief, the Large Intestine also governs all the various daily occurrences of dissatisfaction and disappointment, as well as satisfactions and contentment. Indeed, there is no question that constipation is most unsatisfactory…and that a successful and easy bowel movement can bring a feeling of great relief.

The Large Intestine is very much at play in our state of mind, negative and positive. A happy Large Intestine functioning contributes to a feeling of general optimism whereas a recalcitrant bowel can lead to a deep sense of pessimism and negativity of mind. Keep your colon functioning well, and you may have found one of the key secrets to a happy life.

SPIRITUAL

The spiritual level function of the Large Intestine is no less than the ability to surrender into release and acceptance of the ebb and flow of all conditions. The refrain, "let go and let God" speaks to the high function of Large Intestine at work.

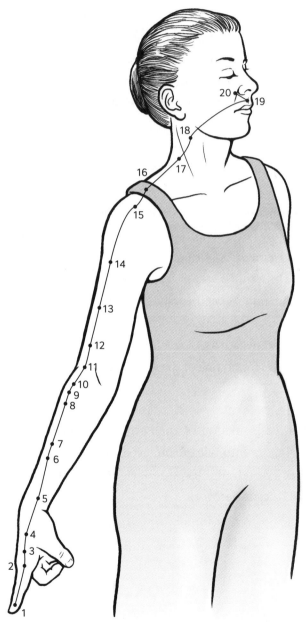

Figure 4: Large Intestine Meridian—Hand Yang Ming.

1. Yang Merchant	11. Pool at the Bend
2. Second Space	12. Elbow Crevice
3. Third Space	13. Arm Five Miles
4. Meeting Valleys	14. Upper Arm
5. Yang Stream (Snuffbox)	15. Shoulder Bone
6. Veering Passage	16. Great Bone
7. Warm Flow	17. Heaven's Tripod
8. Lower Angle	18. Support Prominence
9. Upper Angle	19. Mouth Crevice
10. Arm Three Miles	20. Welcome Fragrance

The Large Intestine Channel Trajectory

From its first point at the tip of the index finger, the Large Intestine makes its way up through the webbing between the thumb and index finger, crosses over and goes through the wrist, up through the elbow, shoulder, neck, and finally into the face ending at the side of the nose, just beside the edge of the nasal opening.

To trace this pathway on yourself, try this easy (if humorous) task: consider how you might wipe a runny nose if you have no handkerchief. You will find that you naturally use the soft, fleshy mound between the root of the forefinger and the thumb to wipe your nose. But you are kneading dough, and your hand is covered with flour so you can't use it! Instead, you wipe your nose with your forearm (I won't tell anyone.) Your nose naturally reaches the fleshy mound of the forearm along the brachio-radialis muscle. But wait, you are actually working under the hood of your car and are greasy up to your elbows! Your nose is itchy and beginning to really run, so you instinctively turn your nose to your shoulder, where it reaches the fleshy front corner.

Congratulations, you have just located your Large Intestine meridian line. All of these places along your arm are directly on the flow of the Large Intestine channel. Once you've done this exercise, you'll never forget the location of the Large Intestine's energy flow in the arm.

We have already been introduced to Large Intestine 1, Yang Merchant, at the end of the index finger. The merchant image helps us understand the place of this meridian in the management of exchange with the outer world. Lung and Large Intestine together make up our border. We need our border to know who we are as distinct from others; to survive we must also interact with others across this border. The border's nature gives rise to the many transactions of our daily life. In this context, consider the many uses of the index finger, the Large Intestine meridian's origin. This finger is the one we use when we are pointing something out to others and when we want to emphasize a detail. In this, we see the aspect of the Large Intestine that governs perfectionism: getting things correct down to the last detail. The index finger points the way.

The meridian continues up the index finger through two points at the knuckle and then we find a major point, 4, Meeting Valleys in the soft mound of flesh just before the root of the thumb. This could well be called the "facial tissue" point, however Meeting Valleys has many functions beyond simply wiping the nose. Among its many uses, it provides relief from the pain of toothache, sinus headache, constipation and diarrhea, and general well-being. The name is provocative and conjures images of the mountain pass where two valleys join, each leading down to opposite sides of the mountain. In order for there to be fair trade, the pass must remain functional and clear. This point is used to maintain clarity and facilitate smooth exchange.

If you should find yourself in the unfortunate position of being constipated, having a headache, or in the dentist's chair, I encourage you to hold this point for a sense of relief. While you hold it, apply steady deep pressure to the point where you really feel the point, and breathe long, steady, slow, deep breaths. Once mastered, the art of accessing the qi flow in the meridian system will give you powerful tools for supporting well-being. This point is an excellent access point to help connect you with the pathway.

From Meeting Valleys, we travel over the thumb joint, up the forearm along the radius bone, and onto the brachio-radialis muscle, called the "carpenter's muscle." If you make the action of gripping a hammer and hammering, you will see this muscle bulge up. At a point on the belly of this muscle three finger-widths distal to the elbow crease, we find Large Intestine 10, Arm Three Miles. (This is likely the point you found earlier when your hands were covered with flour and you went to swipe your nose on your forearm.) As the name implies, Arm Three Miles is a point used for endurance and stamina. Working this point will help you maintain your grip and go that extra mile. Implicit in this definition are the functions of holding on to people and things or letting them go when the time is right. This is a major part of guiding the ship of your life in an artful and effective way.

Continuing on, the meridian flows through the elbow joint and up the arm along the humerus to the corner of the shoulder, where we find Large Intestine 15, Shoulder Bone. This location on the body evokes images of keeping your shoulder to the grindstone. Fortitude and perseverance are hallmarks of this point and this meridian. To have intestinal fortitude has long been noted as a virtue of those who have the guts to carry on even in the face of adversity. And this point, Shoulder Bone, speaks not just to the strength of the shoulder to bear burdens (there's another meridian and shoulder point that has that responsibility), but the rather to the directionality with which we aim our shoulder accurately to cut through the obstacles on the way to our goals.

The meridian now crosses the shoulder at the clavicular-acromial joint, continues over the great trapezius, and through the neck, passing through the sterno-cleido mastoid muscle. It crosses the jaw at the angle of the mandible and ends at the corner of the nose, Large Intestine 20, Welcome Fragrance. To effectively stimulate this point, place the pad of any finger in the depression just lateral to the nostril and under the edge of the bone found there. Angle the finger away from the nose. Now lean your head forward, resting the natural weight of your head on your finger. You will feel an opening of the sinuses with this action. Take a deep breath and smell the roses. The point is the last point on the Large Intestine surface pathway and clearly relates this function to the olfactory sense. Here we can see the strong relationship between smell and our sense of place in the world, yet another example of the way in which we define ourselves in relation to the world around us, a key function of this channel.

Chapter 3

Fulfilling Needs and Wants

In this chapter we explore the Stomach and Spleen channels and their functions in body, heartmind, and spirit. These lines constitute the Tai Yin and Yang Ming aspects of the Earth elemental force and are located in the legs on the front of the body.

Stomach Meridian

Foot Yang Ming

The original name for this channel of energy, the name Foot Yang Ming describes the nature of the energy of this channel, and where it lies on the body. This is the sunlight yang energy as it expresses out through the feet, particularly as it flows from the eyes down through the jaw, throat, breast, belly, thigh, shin, ankle, and out through the second toe. The Stomach is the Foot Yang Ming organ network of the body.

Earth Element

Earth is the term given to the elemental quality of cycles and nourishment. Also attributed to groundedness, sustenance, and the ever-present holding power of gravity. The Stomach organ network is the yang energy of Earth, expressing itself through appetite control and the acquisition of whatever is needed to sustain life. Practically, it is the food we eat. Metaphorically it relates to anything and everything that sustains us through life including contact with loved ones, in addition to nourishing activities that engage our whole being—body, heartmind, and spirit. Earth is the primordial ground upon which we stand, from which we are formed and to which we return.

7 to 9 am

This time of day most commonly correlates to the "breakfast" time of day. It is the start of the day where we first take in food as fuel, building the foundation for our daily activities.

Key Functions

Appetite, hunger, desire/fulfillment, digestion/ingestion of food, maturation

Affirmation

I know what I want and need, and I know how to get it.

The Stomach channel of Foot Yang Ming is the yang aspect of Earth in the body, and it follows a pathway that runs from the eyes to the foot. In a word, it is all about appetite. All living beings have this fundamental function—we all share the necessity that is going out into the world and acquiring whatever is needed to sustain life. When considering the Stomach channel, certainly look at the basic level of the need for proper nutritious food, but also consider all the levels of need and fulfillment within our lives. We strive to be fed in many ways: mentally, emotionally, physically, and spiritually. When someone has a good appetite, they possess a certain zest for life. When appetite dominates too much we see lustful, greedy abandon, and in its absence is wasting away. To understand the full range of Stomach functioning, we need to look at ways in which an organism orients itself toward whatever it seeks for nourishment and sustenance, as well as actions taken to fulfill the acquisition and processing of the desired item, information, or intent. Below we draw out in some detail a wide range of functions characteristic of the Stomach channel.

Key Characteristics of the Functional Range of the Stomach Channel

PHYSICAL

The stomach is the organ that first receives the food we eat, taking the process of digestion forward by breaking down the food. The Stomach channel governs this function and all the related functional aspects of the digestive tract's "tubing." The inner lining of the gut and its many layers of smooth muscle as well as the action of peristalsis (a wavelike series of muscular contractions that move food in the digestive tract) are comprised of a series of ringlike muscles. The Stomach channel governs the opening and closing action of the ring muscles all along the line of the alimentary canal.

In addition to digestive functions, Stomach channel energy is involved in the reproductive system as well. The Foot Yang Ming aspect is particularly related to selection and suitability of a mate, issues of taste, compatibility, and satisfaction. Subsequent questions of fertility and reproductive ability as well as maturity all co-mingle energetically in the realm of the Stomach's role of management. In the case of reproduction, the phrase "another mouth to feed" serves as an example of the Stomach's place in this great task. By extension, the Stomach channel's functions include mammillary glands and the delivery of mother's milk through lactation. Any mastitis or blockage of lactation can be attributed to a blockage in the qi of the Stomach channel.

Psychological, Emotional

By extending the physical action metaphorically into the psychological and emotional realms we can see that Stomach channel has much to do with our urges and motivations caused by hunger and emptiness, needs and wants. These express themselves as nourishment issues, and worthiness issues.

There is a common concern that many people face called the "nourishment barrier." The feeling of a lack of self-worth deeply affects a person's ability to actually take in nourishment.

On the other end of the spectrum, we find the motivators that are eagerness and the desire to seize opportunities. Recalling the Stomach channel's affirmation, we must now make the distinction between needs and wants. You may *want* a new TV, but you *need* clean water. Actually, the making of these distinctions is ruled by another organ network; the Stomach itself is only concerned with the hunger and fulfillment of that hunger, however it may express itself.

Within the Stomach channel we can find the very down-to-earth qualities of lustiness, earthiness, a love of fun, cheerfulness, and confidence. These attitudes can also veer into stubborn, obsessive, or compulsive qualities as well as brooding, chewing, and stewing over all manner of things.

The behavior can show up in many ways, from the parent who is constantly caught up in concerns related to their children's well-being, to the inventor who is constantly worrying about the various details involved in bringing their vision into fruition. Any way you dwell upon a thing and go over and over it in your mind is within the purview of the Stomach channel.

There are few things we do more regularly than feed our belly. And as soon as we are full we leave the table a little bit hungry, wondering about what the next meal might be. Of course, when concerned with your own nourishment, there is a natural human condition that arises where you also find yourself concerned about the nourishment of others.

Anyone who has ever prepared a pot luck dish will know well that feeling of hoping that it will be well received and satisfying. Our concern about others caring for what we created for them is matched by our concern for what they create and feed us.

Arising here is the very human emotion of sympathy and worry, deep expressions of concern for how others feel, and vice versa.

What I've described here can be considered to culminate in the maturation process. Things mellow with time, age and mature, come to fruition.

All the things in life that move along the continuum—from seed to plant to flower to fruit to seed—and all the feelings associated with each stage of the journey are within the realm of Stomach channel energy.

SPIRITUAL

Ultimately, the spiritual level of Stomach is the realization of a deep and satisfying fulfillment, being at peace with what is. It involves an awareness of the cyclical nature of things and a certain cultivated ability to take things in stride.

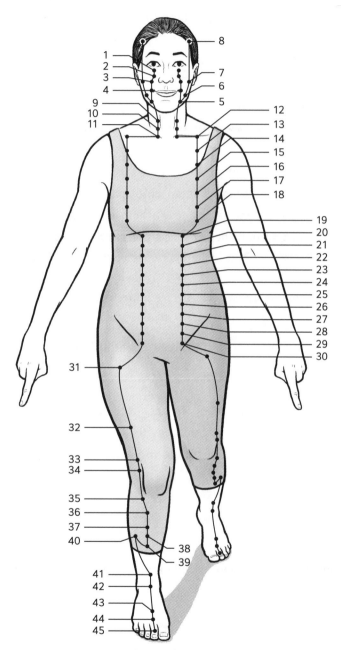

Figure 5: Stomach Meridian—Foot Yang Ming.

1. Tear Receptacle	24. Slippery Flesh Gate
2. Four Whites	25. Celestial Pivot
3. Great Crevice	26. Outer Mound
4. Earth Granary	27. The Great
5. Great Welcome	28. Water Passage
6. Jaw Bone	29. Return
7. Below the Joint	30. Qi Thoroughfare
8. Head Bound	31. Thigh Gate
9. Welcome Human	32. Crouching Rabbit
10. Water Prominence	33. Yin Market
11. Adobe of Qi	34. Ridge Mound
12. Empty Basin	35. Calf's Nose
13. Qi Door	36. Leg Three Miles
14. Storehouse	37. Upper Great Hall
15. Room Divider	38. Ribbon Passage Way
16. Breast Window	39. Lower Great Hall
17. Breast Center	40. Bountiful Bulge
18. Breast Root	41. Stream Divide
19. Not Contained	42. Rushing Yang
20. Supporting Fitness	43. Sunken Valley
21. Beam Gate	44. Inner Courtyard
22. Pass Gate	45. Severe Mouth
23. Supreme Unity	

———+——+———

The Stomach Channel Trajectory

At the point just lateral to the opening of the sinus cavity, the energy of the Large Intestine dissipates, and the one meridian goes inside to re-emerge just under the eye at the first point related to the Stomach function. Here the energy of our appetite and our urge to its fulfillment first manifests on the surface of the body.

In order to appreciate the location of the Stomach meridian on the body, we ask the question, "Can you tell if someone is hungry just by looking at them?" The outward signs of hunger are few. Ultimately, it's really impossible to know that someone is hungry until they say something about it or take actions that clearly indicate their hunger. Those actions, at least for sighted individuals, turn out to be "looking" for food. (How many times have you caught yourself opening the refrigerator or cabinet to peer into the contents to "see" whatever there is to eat?) Here's the clue for the Stomach meridian's opening point on the body's surface: the first point is just below the eyeball, above the lower orbital ridge of the eye socket, directly in alignment with the pupil. Stomach 1, Tear Receptacle, conjures images of a hungry child with one great big tear rolling down from the center of the eye.

From the eye, the meridian travels down the face past the nose, where we smell the food, then into the jaw, where we chew the food, then up to the temple, where we think about the food. Stomach 8, Head Bound, lies here on the superior border of the temporalis muscle. If you place your hands on the sides of your temples and chew, you will feel the action of this muscle. The name "Head Bound" speaks to the way in which our thoughts regarding our needs and wants can take up the whole of our minds, going round and round and round. It is a primary indicator of Stomach meridian functions in action.

We often place our forefingers just here when pondering something of some complexity. And speaking of the stomach, if it's food quality we are pondering, there is much to consider—flavor, quality, origin, preparation. Should the food's taste and quality agree with us, we add it to our diet; if not, we reject it. Really, we do a lot of thinking about food: on one end of the spectrum are the tremendous amounts of research and philosophy that go into our dietary choices, on the other end is our instinct to see food and eat it. The Head Bound point relates to the former approach.

On its way down the throat, the Stomach channel passes through Stomach 9, Welcome Human, also known as Man's Prognosis. Here the carotid artery beats out its faithful rhythm, supporting the good function of the brain. This is a master pulse point for checking the body's status, often the first place a person's life signs are checked after a traumatic accident. Runners check their pulse rate here mid-workout. It's an excellent point for prognosticating, and one of the key prognosticators of good health is a good appetite, hence the name "Man's Prognosis" here on the Stomach meridian in the front of the throat.

From here the meridian continues down the throat. When it reaches the clavicle, it jogs laterally to the mammallary line. It then drops below the collarbone, traversing down the breasts and through the nipple, the source of our first food. Just below the breast it veers back toward the midline where it passes down through the digestive area. At the level of the navel we find Stomach 25, Celestial Pivot, the Large Intestine "alarm point." Chinese medicine teaches us that the Stomach rules the Intestine. It is often said that you are what you eat, but this is not exactly true— what's true is that you are what you don't eliminate. The intestines play a major part of separating nutrition from waste. As such what we eat and how we eat it is the first step in the process that ends with what we integrate as nutrition, and what we eliminate as waste. The relationship between Stomach and Large Intestine plays out at Stomach 25.

Below the navel, the meridian passes through the region of the reproductive organs. As with food, we also have appetites for intimacy and sexual activity. Here the need and fulfillment cycle is evident, though often the source of great challenges and consternation. It all coalesces in Stomach 30, Qi Thoroughfare, at the lateral edge of the pubic bone. The qi flows like a great river through this major point, passing from upper body to our lower body.

From the pubic region, the meridian moves laterally and descends through the strong support muscle of the thigh, the vastus lateralis, to the knee. Passing laterally past the kneecap and over the head of the tibia, the most weight bearing bone in the entire body, it lands in a cavity known as Stomach 36, Leg Three Miles. This point is nearly epic in its significance, holding legendary power and efficacy. It has been used for centuries as a point for general well-being, stamina, and endurance. It is said that when the imperial message runners of Japan and China were fatigued, they would bend over and stimulate this point, allowing them to continue running. "Three Miles" is a euphemism for many miles, and stimulation of this point has long been held as essential self-care for life's long journey.

In bit of folk wisdom, young men are warned in Japan: "Don't marry a woman who does not have moxa scars on Stomach 36!" Moxa is mugwort wool that is burned on the acupoints to send deep, penetrating heat into the body for support of optimal functioning of the system. Scarring moxibustion is a traditional treatment in Japan and China where the moxa wool is burned right down to the skin, leaving a visible scar. In those times, there was obviously less concern for physical appearance and more for robust health. A woman with moxa scars on Stomach 36 would be seen as responsible and concerned for her well-being, knowing how to carry herself. Without these scars, it would imply that she does not know how to take care of herself and would overburden any poor bloke who might marry her.

Another aspect important to point out here is that from Stomach 36 onward to Stomach 45 at the second toe, we can see a pathway in the leg that is very similar to the pathway of Large Intestine in the forearm. From the second digit to the Three Mile point in each channel, they run a very similar aspect of the appendage. This similarity underscores the relationship between Stomach and Large Intestine as both being qualities of Yang Ming energy in the body.

The Stomach channel continues down along the lateral aspect of the tibia, the most weight bearing bone in the body. The image of sustenance, endurance, and stamina all can be reflected in this aspect. Crossing the ankle, we find Stomach 41, Stream Divide, or Shoelace Point, deep in the retinacula of the ankle. Found in many places in the body, retinacula are horizontal tendonous sheaths that wrap around the longitudinal muscles and ligaments of the joints, girdling or wrapping around the joints like natural, internal Ace bandages. Deep in the retinacula of the ankle, Stomach 41, Shoelace Point once again demonstrates the key role the Stomach channel plays in supporting the body in holding it all together.

Passing the ankle, the channel then flows down the top of the foot coming to completion in the second toe at Stomach 45, Severe Mouth. This strong name at the extremity of the channel once again links back to the Stomach channel and its relationship to the mouth. The point has clinically been used to stop an epileptic fit, which often presents as a swallowing of the tongue. A severe condition of the mouth, indeed, and deeply related to the Stomach meridian.

All in all, we find that this strong showing of the Stomach channel in the legs demonstrates the key role the Stomach plays in supporting and sustaining our life energy. Note that the second toe (sometimes longer than the big toe) is also a very clear indicator of the direction in which we are headed. We push off of it while taking strides in the direction of our new interest.

This final aspect of the meridian tied together with the entire picture of the location of the Stomach channel illustrates the understanding that the Stomach meridian is deeply related to all the motivations in life that draw us forward. It is the proverbial carrot on the stick that draws us on in pursuit of that which we desire.

Spleen/Pancreas Meridian
Foot Tai Yin

We've explored Tai Yin of the hand as it expresses in the Lung channel. Here we find Tai Yin of the foot expressed as the Spleen channel. Note that the Spleen channel begins in the big toe and rises up to the breast, where it almost joins the Lung channel below the clavicle. And while Spleen tails down into the side ribs to make connection to the Heart channel, the Tai Yin energy carries on into the arms as Lung energy and completes its run in the thumb.

Earth Element

As the Stomach expresses the yang aspect of Earth in the body, the Spleen expresses the yin aspect of Earth. All the elements have a yin and yang expression, and as we explore each system you will see that the yin is the more "dense" organ and the yang is the more "hollow" organ. The lungs and spleen are dense and vascularized, the stomach and large intestine are tubes and holding tanks. With Spleen as an expression of yin Earth, we will see much more involved on the fluid level, the body's moisture and lubricant that keeps things moving through the tubes.

9 to 11 am

This time of day is rich and productive; many people agree that this period is when they get the most done. It is also a clue to the function of Spleen, and difficulties occuring at this time of day can indicate problems with the Spleen function.

Key Functions

Digestive secretions, reproductive hormones

Affirmation

I love sweetness and thrive on nurturing and being nourished.

The Spleen channel of Foot Tai Yin is the yin aspect of Earth, traveling a pathway from the foot to the torso. To understand the functional range of the Spleen channel we need to extend the analogy beyond the spleen organ and include the pancreas. When the Traditional Chinese system was being translated, the term "Spleen" was used and became generally accepted as the name for the channel, though in actuality its range of functioning more closely relates to the pancreas. The Spleen is all about nourishment, digestion, blood sugar levels, and maintaining good working order. As the yin organ of Earth, it holds the position of converting grain into usable energy to meet bodily needs. In this capacity it is deeply related to the quality of the blood; the levels and transportation of nutrient energy throughout the body. It is related to keeping things in their place and keeping things at peace. A healthy Spleen/Pancreas leads us into contentment and satisfaction. When unhealthy, we experience worry, over thinking, discontent, and the like. Let's explore these basic functional features in greater detail.

Key Characteristics of the Functional Range of the Spleen Channel

PHYSICAL

As the yin quality of Earth energy in the body, the Spleen channel is related to fluids of digestion—saliva, gastric bile, and digestive enzymes— in addition to all the fluid mechanisms that break down and gather nutrients and carry them into the bloodstream. The Spleen is concerned with blood sugar, blood sugar levels, and the energy we receive as a result.

Female hormonal fluids and balance of the menstrual cycle, ovulation, and lactation are all governed by Spleen function. The theme of cycles shows up here too: smooth, predictable, and repeated flow is the realm of Spleen function. If there is a disruption in the cycle, or things are out of place, the Spleen's qi is compromised.

The very flesh of the body is also the physical manifestation of Spleen channel energy in the body. We sometimes pack on a little "winter weight" and shed it off in the summer, again, a natural cycle of things. Women may see weight fluctuate with the menstrual cycle due to what is commonly called water weight. This too is the realm of Spleen. How we hold on to, store, cling, worry over, or otherwise grasp and embrace can show up in the quality of the fleshy weight of the body.

PSYCHOLOGICAL, EMOTIONAL

To seek comfort, pleasure, and ease with all your needs met is a psychological and emotional reflection of Spleen channel energy. Aspects of laziness and lethargy can set in, as can those days where you lie about and indulge yourself as a way of self-nourishment. I never used to let myself have such days, always driven to be on some task; my Spleen energy was being used up. When I finally learned to slow down and take an occasional "couch day," my Spleen became a lot happier.

In those whose Spleens are generally excessive and amped up on a regular basis, we find the habits of overthinking, worrying, and either really thinking things through ... or worrying to death.

Overeating, eating fast, and the "stuff and go" behavior—the typical American fast food kind of lifestyle that eats big, runs fast, and builds big—are maladies that can affect those who have not learned to regulate their Spleen function. Think of America's tall buildings, big cities, high yield activities, 24/7/365, burn, burn, burn, go, go, go. They portray a way the Spleen channel can express itself, and of course when that proves to be a problem, the concomitant problems of obesity, disordered eating, obsession, compulsion, and addiction follow.

Finally, let's consider our dear sweet tooth and any and all other cravings for that matter as expressions of Spleen channel energy. It is the aspect of ourselves that is ever wanting, longing, striving to fulfill, and fill that deep hole inside. On the upside, it can be balanced ambition toward a goal we care about that continues to drive us forward in a sustainable way. But it can also consume us like gold fever, turning us into a dysfunctional mess.

SPIRITUAL

Here we take a long view and see that the cycles of life, time, and tide ultimately settle all things. We arrive at the satisfaction of sufficiency—enough, no more, no less—and sustainability over the long term for all concerned.

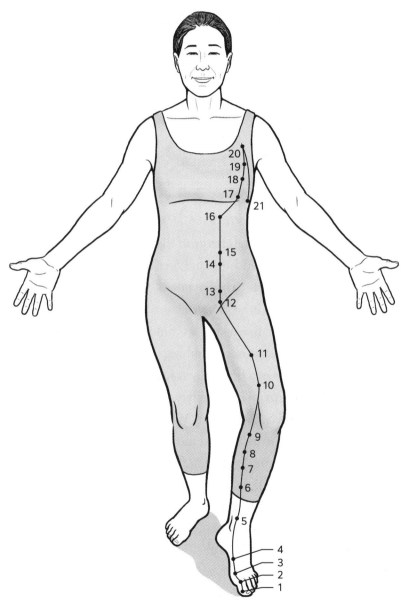

Figure 6: Spleen/Pancreas Meridian—Foot Tai Yin.

1. Hidden White	12. Rushing Gate
2. Great Metropolis	13. Abode of the Yin Organs
3. Supreme White	14. Abdomen Knot
4. Grandfather Grandson	15. Great Horizontal
5. Trade Winds Mound	16. Abdomen Sorrow
6. Three Yin Meeting	17. Food Cavity
7. Granary Hole	18. Heavenly Stream
8. Earth's Crux	19. Chest Village
9. Yin Mound Spring	20. Encircling Glory
10. Sea of Blood	21. Great Embracement
11. Winnower's Gate	

The Spleen/Pancreas Channel Trajectory

At the tip of the second toe, the energy of the Stomach completes its journey on the body's surface and the one meridian goes inside again only to emerge one toe over at the medial edge of the big toe. Spleen energy begins to show itself. As it is a yin meridian and has a more inward function to play, we find its pathway follows a more intimate arc of the body generally more tender to the touch and responsive to stimulation.

From the big toe, Spleen begins by tracing the edge of the instep and arch of the foot. Just proximal and inferior to the head of the first metatarsal bone we find Spleen 3, Supreme White. This is the source point on the Spleen meridian, and as an antique point it governs the Earth element. The word "white" in the name refers to the color of Metal, invoking the creation cycle relationship of the five elements. Earth engenders Metal, and this point can be used to nourish a deficient Lung pattern.

Next we have Spleen 4, Grandfather Grandson, in the depression just distal and inferior to the head of the first metatarsal bone. Also known as Grandparent Grandchild or Yellow Emperor, this point is the opening point for the Chong Mai, the central vessel. The Chong Mai is said to hold the blueprint for our lives that comes down from our ancestors. It is one of the eight extraordinary vessels and is accessed through Spleen 4. Here we can see a deep relationship between our conditioned and constitutional layers of health; the deep connection between what nourishes us on the surface but also reflects who we are in the world.

From the foot, the Spleen channel crosses over the medial maleolous, up the medial aspect of the leg, following along the posterior aspect of the tibia. This is a deep trough in the body landscape and is often quite sensitive to the touch. Right in this trough, four fingers above the medial maleolous we find Spleen 6, Three Yin Meeting. Here the three yin energies of Tai Yin, Jue Yin, and Shao Yin converge. Profoundly important for our health and well-being, Spleen, Liver, and Kidney energies all manifest here. This is a major point, useful for myriad indications, chief among them womens' reproductive cycle issues and childbirth.

Continuing up this trough we find Spleen 7, Granary Hole; 8, Earth's Crux; and 9, Yin Mound Spring. All are extremely important points for positively affecting digestive activity.

Located in a depression just distal to the head of the tibia in between the medial border of the tibia and the gastrocnemius, Spleen 9, Yin Mound Spring, is used to asses and treat the condition of dampness as it affects the digestive system, particularly the lower abdomen. Dampness is an important pathology, quite common in those with a poor diet that's rich in mucous producing foods like white flour, white sugar, and dairy products. Dampness manifests as a sense of tired heaviness and lethargy and includes a host of maladies related to sluggishness in the body, heartmind, and spirit. The proverbial wet blanket is a perfect image for capturing a picture of dampness. If you or anyone you know suffers from this, you will find Spleen 9 sensitive and painful. Stimulation of this point through exercise, meditation touch, or needling can bring some much-appreciated relief.

Crossing the knee joint, Spleen finds its way into the vastus medialis muscle of the thigh along the medial aspect of the quadriceps. In the head of that muscle just proximal to the knee joint we find Spleen 10, Sea of Blood, effective for menstrual issues and blood sugar challenges. Then just halfway up the thigh along the same muscle we find Spleen 11, Winnower's Gate. I especially love this point and its name because it is so evocative. For those not familiar (and most of us haven't heard the word recently unless we live on a farm), winnowing is the process of sorting the grain from the chaff. In a traditional setting, the winnower would have a large tray filled with grain and chaff. While squatting, the person would throw the grain and chaff into the air with a rhythmic action. The light chaff is borne away on the wind, while the heavier grain falls to be caught again in the winnower's tray. If you squat down and mimic this action, you will find that your elbows naturally find a place to rest on the medial aspect of the thigh, midway between the knee and the groin—this is the Winnower's Gate. The point is used to support the digestive system, and its function of assimilating nutrition from food we intake and eliminating the rest is, in short, winnowing.

Continuing up the thigh and into the abdomen, Spleen crosses over the Stomach meridian and makes its way up the abdominal muscles, lateral to the Stomach flow and four inches off centerline. Several points in the abdomen can all be used to assist the Spleen in its digestive functioning. As the channel enters the chest, it glances sideways to move up lateral to the breast tissue until it arrives at its most superior point—Spleen 20, Encircling Glory, just one inch below Central Treasury, the first point on the Lung channel. This point location is illustrative of the Spleen's close association with Lung, as both are Tai Yin meridians.

After reaching almost to the Lung point, the channel turns and tails down and out toward the side of the body, coming to a close at Spleen 21, Great Embracement, in the sixth intercostal space on the midaxillary line. This is an extremely influential point in the channel system. In addition to being the final point on the Spleen meridian it is also the Great Luo Point, or Connecting Vessel point that links the Spleen to the Heart. In Western parlance we have a saying that recognizes this important connection: "The way to a man's heart is through his stomach." In this case, we adapt the saying slightly: "The path to the heart is through the spleen," in short, whatever nourishes the body nourishes the heartmind as well.

Chapter 4

Higher Truth, Integration and Assimilation, Sovereignty and Order

In this chapter we explore the Heart and Small Intestine channels of qi and their functions in body, heartmind, and spirit. Note that these lines constitute the Shao Yin and Tai Yang aspects of absolute Fire and are located in the body along the back of the arms.

Heart Meridian

Hand Shao Yin

The Shao Yin energies are the body's deep yin energies. The Hand Shao Yin is identified with the heart, the deep and mysterious organ beating steadily at the core of our being. Ultimately, it is the master of everything we embrace at a deep level. The Heart channel of Hand Shao Yin is the full expression of this deep inner aspect of life.

Absolute Fire Element

The absolute Fire element is that quality of light and heat that inspires and transforms, enlightens and informs us at each step of the way. Fire offers heat, light, renewal, and regeneration. It can also sear, burn, cook, and utterly incinerate. The deep truth that resides in the Heart can set us free and can also burn away falsehood, but it is not always the most comfortable task.

11 am to 1 pm

High noon: the hour of truth when shadows are at their shortest. There is nowhere to easily hide at this time of day. Conversely, you may want to find a rock to crawl under for shade and cooling at this time of day.

Key Functions

Personal truth, interpretation, communication, sovereign order

Affirmation

I harmonize with the inner truth in my Heart.

The Heart channel of Hand Shao Yin is the yin aspect of the absolute Fire in the body, and it follows a trajectory that begins deep in the axilla (armpit) and ends in the pinky finger. It is referred to as the Supreme Sovereign Emperor or Ruler of the Realm and as such is charged with the duty of holding the divine vision for the body's life. It rests deep in the chest with the most protection from direct outside contact, and yet in its position at the core of our being it has a guiding influence over our every action. Anatomical science has established that the heart is not directed by the nervous system in any way. Its highly specialized cells know their job without the need for stimulation from the central nervous system. Of course it carries and pumps blood through the body; it is also considered to be where the spirit resides. Many speak to heart's role in life. "He wears his heart on his sleeve," "She plays her cards close to her chest," "She has a heart of gold," "My heart is in the work," "I'm living my heart's desire."

These are all expressions that hint at what the Heart channel's functional range is all about. What follows is a description of the Heart channel's key characteristics, a most auspicious set of functions in human life.

Key Characteristics of the Functional Range of the Heart Channel

PHYSICAL

The fundamental rhythm of the heartbeat accompanies every moment of daily life. At its most physical level, the Heart channel governs the diastolic and systolic pressure of blood flowing in and out of the heart, both in timing and volume and the intricate way in which this rhythm subtly conducts the affairs of the body's every aspect.

By extension, the Heart channel governs the body's blood and blood vessels from the major arteries and veins to the capillaries. Any signs or symptoms arising from the functioning of the arteries and veins—from the flow of blood to the pressure in the vessels—can all be addressed through the Heart channel.

The most necessary function of perspiration in the regulation of body temperature is also related to the Heart channel function. This key function of maintaining and sustaining body temperature is closely governed by the Fire element. The Heart channel gets extra support from other channels in this most essential aspect of balance.

Interestingly, the Heart channel also governs the functioning of the tongue and speech. Because the Heart is directly related to the truth, all uses of the tongue and speech come under the direction of the Heart. To be in alignment with your truth is to never utter a false word. Sometimes you may find that you need to hide your truth because it is dangerous to speak it. Or you may find yourself lying or "speaking with forked tongue." These are all related to the very physical act of speaking. One final link between the Heart and speech can be observed in many cases of cardiac arrest: slurring of the speech is one major symptom.

Psychological, Emotional

The understanding of the Heart channel's core, physical function causes us to consider the deep work that is inner reflection and soul searching. These are at the very foundation of emotional feeling and intimacy. When we are in touch with our Heart's true nature and able to express it in good company, we are given access to the joy and laughter that can release daily life's tensions and stresses. When the Heart channel functions at full capacity a deep, internally courageous aspect of great worth shows itself.

Spiritual

At the spiritual level Heart channel keeps us in our compassion, truth, kindness, and joy. It opens us to transcendent bliss in which we move beyond duality and become all embracing.

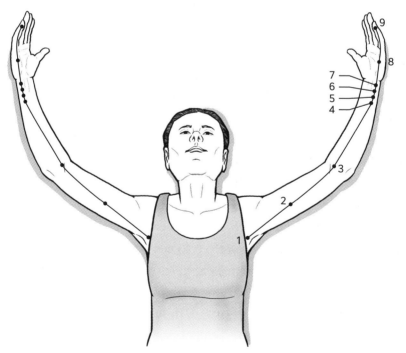

Figure 7: Heart Meridian—Hand Shao Yin.

1. Highest Spring	6. Yin Cleft
2. Cyan Spirit	7. Spirit Gate
3. Lesser Seas	8. Lesser Palace
4. Spirit Path	9. Lesser Rushing
5. Penetrating the Interior	

The Heart Channel Trajectory

As Spleen energy completes its section of the cycle, the one meridian goes inside to reemerge nearby at the center of the axilla, the center of the armpit, the first point on the Heart meridian. Heart 1, Highest Spring, is a point for which direct stimulation is forbidden in the ancient texts. Indeed, the entire meridian is often never treated directly but rather affected through stimulation of all other channels which exist to support the highest truth of the Heart, its sovereign ruler. The Heart is considered the supreme commander of the body, and like the emperor leads through example and divine connection rather than through actual effort. The actions of the realm are to be carried out by lesser ministers, leaving the sovereign to weighty matters such as philosophy and the divine purposes of life. Heart 1, Highest Spring, connotes the springing forth of the most high and divine waters to nourish the people and the realm with wisdom and order. Of all the spring points on the body (of which there are many), this point is also closest to the heavens, physically speaking.

Soft and vulnerable yet strong and stable, Heart energy runs through the most tender region, just under the biceps where the brachial pulse can be felt. Here at Heart 2, Cyan Spirit, the presence of energy at the surface is most readily discovered; even a light touch on others will send reverberations through your own being. Perhaps the expression to "wear your heart on your sleeve" reflects this understanding of the placement of the Heart channel on the surface of the arm. In many of the world's religious traditions we also see the raising up of the arms, actually opening the

Heart energy to the heavens, as an expression of opening the Heart to the divine. From the brachial plexus, the Heart energy takes a course from the inside of the elbow along the ulna to the wrist.

At the wrist we find Heart 7, Spirit Gate. This point is critical in treating insomnia, dream-disturbed sleep, and schizophrenia. The Heart as emperor is seen as exemplar of Fire, the element of light and truth, awareness and wakefulness. When the yang aspect of our fire is overactive and the yin aspect is deficient, we are restless, dream-filled, and cannot sleep peacefully. Too much "burning of the candle at both ends", will eventually lead us to "burn out," and our Hearts will be exhausted. Heart 7, Spirit Gate may be useful in restoring our connection to an inexhaustible universal resource, giving our own Heart a much-needed rest.

The Heart channel continues across the palm and ends at the pinky finger, ending at Heart 9, Lesser Rushing. This name reflects the understanding that the ends of the fingers are seen as points from which our qi energy emanates, perhaps overromanticized in the Star Wars saga when blue forks of force lightning emanate from the emperor's fingertips. And the word "lesser" in the name refers to both the little finger and the Heart as the Shao Yin, or lesser yin energetic function in the body, heartmind, and spirit. The distinction of lesser yin is often confusing to our Western way of thinking that perceives "lesser" as a diminutive adjective. Rather, it is useful to consider the adage "less is more" and see the extreme yin virtue of the Heart as being at its strongest when at rest.

Stories from old China link the pinky finger to our deepest inner passions, hence the naming of this smallest digit as the "finger of passion." Accordingly, the punishment for crimes of passion was to have this digit amputated. If you met someone who had this finger removed, you would know that person had violated the sanctity of an intimate boundary in an unlawful way in the past. It is a powerful finger in its own distinct way and speaks to the refinement that comes from the feelings of the heart.

Small Intestine Meridian

Hand Tai Yang

The Hand Tai Yang is greater yang energy as it expresses through the Small Intestine channel organ network. A bright and vigorous yang, it is the height of the active principle and has the capacity for strong, direct, and impassioned action.

Absolute Fire Element

The Heart channel carries forth the yin aspect of absolute Fire and the Small Intestine is its yang counterpart. The strong Fire here can express itself in bold strokes and fiery action. One can liken the Small Intestine's absolute Fire quality to the sword of truth, the blade that can cut through the BS and tell it like it is without fear or anxiety.

1 to 3 pm

The height of the day represents this culmination of yang energy. This is the day's last hurrah before the encroaching night with its lengthening shadows that bring back the yin of night once more.

Key Functions

Discernment, judgment, assimilation, absorption

Affirmation

I see what is true and what is false, and I keep only what is true for me.

The Small Intestine channel of Hand Tai Yang is the yang aspect of absolute Fire and follows a trajectory that runs from the hands to the face. It is known as the minister in charge of separating the pure from the impure. When we look at this on the physical level, we can clearly see the small intestine with its many fine cilia sweeping the digestive tract, separating nutrients from our dietary intake for absorption directly into the bloodstream, while passing the waste to the large intestine for processing.

On the mental and emotional levels, we must also separate out the important from the unimportant. In our age of information overload, the Small Intestine is acutely tasked with sorting this mass of information and distilling the essence for use. It calls upon our faculties of discernment and higher judgment to be finely honed. When it is in distress, we are overwhelmed and may make bad choices as a result of being easily misled or overly skeptical. What follows is an overview of the range of characteristics the Small Intestine channel governs.

Key Characteristics of the Functional Range of the Small Intestine Channel

PHYSICAL

According to Chinese medical classics, the Small Intestine channel has the primary function in the human body of separating the pure from the impure. The small intestine organ is adjacent to the stomach in the alimentary canal. It receives the digesta (food that has been transformed through mastication and the stomach's action into the liquid slurry passed to the small intestine for processing) directly from the stomach and performs the vital role of nutrient extraction. Its ingenuity lies in its ability to separate the nutrition from the waste with thousands of tiny cilia, hair-like structures lining its interior walls. The cilia absorb the nutrients and pass them through the lining of the small intestine to the hepatic portal vein, the blood vessel that draws the nutrient from the small intestine to carry it through the blood directly to the liver. Blood cells are also created here, and so we see Small Intestine channel playing a vital role in building blood, the liquid fuel of the body.

The process of separating the pure from the impure is the metabolic fire that continually breaks down, converts, and transforms food we have eaten into the nutritional components necessary for feeding all the cellular activity within the body. It is known as "digestive fire" or *agni* in the Ayurvedic medicine of India. Indigestion is therefore the lack of digestive fire; intestinal inflammation would be an excess of digestive fire. All manner of bowel concerns like diverticulitis, leaky gut, ulcerative colitis, and so on are governed by the Small Intestine channel and can be treated via points on the channel.

Beyond this direct relationship to the digestion of food, the Small Intestine channel also concerns itself with the digestion of all sorts of stimuli. Of particular note is the processing of auditory information in the process known as selective hearing. Within a field of auditory information we can select whatever is important to hear and pay attention only to that. Selective hearing is also sometimes called "cocktail party hearing"; all around you are a hundred ongoing conversations, but you only track the one in which you are engaged. Your ear is an extension of Small Intestine function in this way. Like the small intestine, the inner ear also has thousands of cilia that register the various sounds of the environment. From a vast field of noise, it can pick out the important from the unimportant.

Psychological, Emotional

Building metaphorically upon its physical functions, on the psychological level we find the Small Intestine channel busy with the task of prioritizing and being focused on goals. The ability to distinguish the important from the superfluous is used in an ongoing and rapid manner, repeating throughout the day. The process of prioritizing and sorting through all the various stimuli and choices before us is a necessity when living in a complex world, and the ongoing nature of this task leads to the development of qualities of determination. In a case where Small Intestine energies are strong we see it as determination to the bitter end; when weak, we see a complete lack of determination and an inability to stay focused and follow through on tasks, promises, or commitments.

Determination and discrimination are quite individual-based; accordingly, the Small Intestine has an important role to play in self-analysis as well. It governs the ability to truly look at and listen to oneself, the discovery of our own inner truth. For instance, a common struggle is the conversation between the heart and the head: if your heart holds a particular truth about yourself, your passion, what you truly love, but your head is filled with ideas that somehow what you love is wrong, bad, or simply unimportant in the world, the battle between the two rages. The Small Intestine channel performs the vitally important role of supporting communication and ultimately reconciliation between your head and your heart, as well as between your heart and the hearts of others. The adage about wearing your heart on your sleeve gets a little rewrite here—ideally you wear your Small Intestine on your sleeve! The Heart itself remains sovereign and protected from direct exposure to the sensory overload of the world in which it finds itself.

With all its heavy tasks and serious duties of winnowing down the myriad choices to come up with exactly the right path for you, it may be surprising that the Small Intestine also plays a vital role in your sense of humor. The ability to laugh out loud is directly governed by the Small Intestine, and in a world with so many switchbacks, tricksters, and blind alleys amid the foibles and vagaries of natural consequences, you are in for a hard, hard ride if you aren't equipped with a good sense of humor. In many ways, the gift of laughter can be sanity's safety valve. Consider how it is often received through the gift of time: "One day we'll look back on this and laugh" is a comment often made in the midst of moments with great weight and consequence. The Small Intestine is concerned with the distinction here as well.

SPIRITUAL

On the spiritual level, the Small Intestine channel can be summed up as the faculty for better judgment. When faced with a multitude of concerns, the spiritual task at hand is really the manner in which you go about choosing the highest and best path that will most serve your deepest truth. And when you misstep, a healthy Small Intestine channel will grant you the spiritual ability to forgive yourself (and others) and even laugh at your foibles.

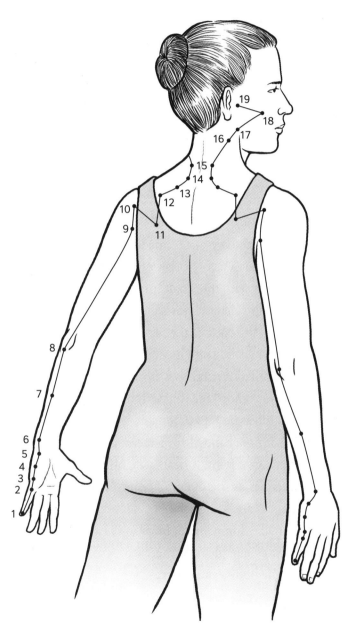

Figure 8: Small Intestine Meridian—Hand Tai Yang.

1. Lesser Marsh	11. Heavenly Gathering
2. Front Valley	12. Grasping the Wind
3. Back Stream	13. Crooked Wall
4. Wrist Bone	14. Outer Shoulder Transport
5. Yang Valley	15. Middle Shoulder Transport
6. Support the Aged	16. Heavenly Window
7. Upright Branch	17. Divine Appearance
8. Small Sea	18. Cheek Bone Hole
9. Correct Shoulder	19. Palace of Hearing
10. Upper Arm Transport	

Small Intestine Channel Trajectory

The Heart energy finishes here at the medial aspect of the little finger, and our one meridian takes a tiny step to the lateral aspect of the same digit to begin its journey with the Small Intestine energy. From the pinky finger, the Small Intestine channel flows along the "karate chop" edge of the fifth metacarpal on the back of the hand. The Small Intestine's function is to sort through anything sent its way via the Stomach, separate out the nutrition for assimilation, and pass on the waste. One might see in the action of the "karate chop" the function of slicing through whatever presents itself. Small Intestine 3, Back Stream, is found on the karate chop edge of the hand, just under the fifth metacarpal bone, just proximal to the metacarpal/phalangeal joint. It bears a significant relationship to all the body's yang energies as the opening point for the governing vessel. The governing vessel is also called the Sea of Yang, running directly up the center of the spinal column. Small Intestine as a Tai Yang vessel is the most superficial of yang energies and therefore provides a ready gateway into the entirety of the body's yang energy. Separating the pure from the impure is considered a yang task.

Leaving the hand and crossing over the wrist, we find Small Intestine 6, Supporting the Aged, in the bony cleft on the radial side of the styloid process of the ulna. This point and its name are related to steady control of the hand, as motor skills become shakier with age. Again, the relationship between steadiness of the hand and the ability to discern between what is useful and what is useless is reflected here.

The channel then travels along the ulnar surface of the arm to the funny bone point at the elbow, Small Intestine 8, Small Sea. The name is somewhat enigmatic and refers to the classical understanding that qi runs deep at this point and enters the Small Intestine like a river flowing into the sea. In terms of physical actions and uses for this point, we might practice the gesture of elbowing our way through the crowd. Imagine you are at a sports or music event and want to make your way forward to get a good, clear view of the action. The Small Intestine's job is knowing how to discern the best from the rest in order to attain clarity.

The channel continues up the posterior edge of the triceps to the juncture of the arm and shoulder. Here we find Small Intestine 9, Correct Shoulder, deep in the belly of the teres minor muscle, one of four muscles that make up the rotator cuff. These four muscles have the job of keeping the arm properly attached to the shoulder, so the point name reinforces the idea of keeping this joint in correct working order. Perhaps the ancients didn't think of it this way, but correct bearing in the shoulders could be considered related to the Small Intestine performing its official task. Another gesture that wields this aspect of our body can be seen in the action of the judge's arm that brings the gavel down to bring order to the courtroom. In addition to enforcing order and conduct in an unruly courtroom, the judge pounds the gavel at the pronouncement of the sentence. Once again we see the relation to the Small Intestine's function, discerning good from bad. Indeed, discernment and maintaining order hold a place of great esteem and lofty respect in society.

From Small Intestine 9 the channel continues its journey into the shoulder blade. In the center of the sub-scapular fossa we find Small Intestine 11, Heavenly Gathering, also known as Center of Heaven. We smile as we think of this as the place where our angel wings are attached when on Judgment Day it is determined that we have led an exemplary life. Here again is Small Intestine's discrimination faculty being recognized once more, as well as the channel's Fire quality. The most yang of the elements, Fire is most closely associated with transcendent reflection.

Here in the wings we also find Small Intestine 12, Grasping the Wind, at the very top of the shoulder blade. In our avian cousins, this bone is the leading edge of the wing that takes the bird into flight. Here we grasp and ride the winds of life.

From the wings, the channel crosses the neck and the jaw to the peak of the cheekbone. Small Intestine 18, Cheek Bone Hole, rests right at this crest of the cheek; a high and well defined cheekbone signifies a certain refinement in the human form. From Cheek Bone Hole, the channel follows the line of the zygomatic arch back to the ear, where with an open jaw we find a small depression between the tragus and mandibular joint. At this point on the Small Intestine channel we have direct access to that vital faculty of selective hearing at Small Intestine 19, Palace of Hearing. In addition to being useful in treating all manner of hearing disorders, the word *palace* in the name evokes imagery of a throne or court. And when used as a noun, *hearing* refers to courtroom proceedings. In a hearing, two sides of a case are presented, and the judge must discern which side is lawful and has merit and which is false and must be ruled against. Once again, the Small Intestine function of discernment is illustrated here, and the ear is directly connected to the gavel of justice's pounding.

The Small Intestine channel has now run its course, giving way to the next channel of energy flow, the Bladder channel, beginning at the eye's inner tear duct.

Chapter 5

Flight from Danger, Life and Death Instincts

In this chapter we explore the Bladder and Kidney channels of qi and their functions in body, heartmind, and spirit. Note that these lines constitute the Shao Yin and Tai Yang aspects of the Water elemental force and are located in the body along the back and the back of the legs. The Kidney also travels up the front of the torso, quite close to the body's midline.

Bladder Meridian

Foot Tai Yang

The Tai Yang energy of the hand has connected to the Tai Yang energy of the foot, and we find the strong yang energy flowing from the eyes up over the crown of the head and down the back body all the way to the pinky toe. This is energetically the most yang area of the body, the broad back, the most exposed to the world, and also the one part of the body most difficult to look at directly. We can only observe our own Tai Yang from within using our inner eyes and felt sense for life.

Water Element

The yang aspect of the Water element is expressing itself here in this channel. In water we see a strong yet patient presence. Water can be still as a mountain lake or wild and mad as a raging storm. Water is vital and mysterious, soft and powerful, holds all things, and can be deep and unfathomable. Like Fire, it holds us in fascination and mystery for its powerful and essential place in nature.

3 to 5 pm

The period in the afternoon has long been known as a transitional time. The day itself is dwindling, the shadows lengthening, and the night heralded. The Bladder channel sits here and gives us the capacity to nap or take tea or a coffee break. Whatever we choose to do, we are finding the strength to power through the rest of the day.

Key Functions

Drive, purification, autonomic nervous system

Affirmation

I drive myself forward, keeping an eye on my back.

The Bladder channel of Foot Tai Yang is the yang aspect of Water found in the body, and it follows a pathway from the eyes to the feet. On the physical level the bladder is seen as the organ that stores and eliminates the body's fluid waste. Examining this function, we can see how it is representative of the faculties of flexibility and capacity. When we reflect upon the experience of bladder functioning, we recognize urgency and drive as fundamental aspects.

Few urges are stronger than the one to urinate when necessary. And the capacity to "hold it" until arriving at a proper facility is a skill we learn over time. As infants we pee anywhere, and as we grow up we must learn to manage this function properly. The Bladder channel thus represents any area of our lives where we must manage ourselves and also focus our intention and move forward with strength and power and wisdom. The channel itself runs down the back, and as such represents our past, all that is behind us. It is also our unconscious, aspects of ourselves that are most difficult to view. Try as you might, you cannot see your back by turning your head.

Only with mirrors or the help of friends and inward looking can we get a glimpse of this aspect of our being. The Bladder meridian is pervasive as well, featuring points along it relating to all the body's functional systems. Traveling as it does along the spine, it relates to all the enervations of the central nervous system and is therefore central in all nervous system functions. More details of its functions are found in the descriptions that follow.

Key Characteristics of the Functional Range of the Bladder Channel

PHYSICAL

The Bladder channel is named after the urinary bladder organ, but its range of function in the physical body goes way beyond the tasks of storing and releasing the body's liquid waste. That storing and releasing function can serve as a metaphor for what we might call the body's capacity and deep inner motivations. How much can you hold? How long can you hold it? When you've got to do it, you get it done! It's all pre-wired and happens as a nearly instinctual and primary function, allowing us to go about the business of living.

Here we find ourselves analyzing the Bladder channel's governance of the autonomic nervous system, all those myriad nervous system functions throughout the brain, spinal cord, and all the interconnected synapses of the sensory and motor neuron system.

The autonomic nervous system is responsible for all the feedback loops and automatic responses as well as the intelligence of all the systems of the body that perform their tasks without the need for conscious intervention, knowledge, or consent.

Within the purview of automated tasks is the entire panoply of human growth and development. Of particular interest to the Bladder channel are the bones, the many small and large rigid tissues of the body comprising the skeletal system. Here we see the formation of structure and again the body's capacity to maintain integrity in the midst of physical stress and strain as well as the effects of those stresses and strains on the skeletal structure.

PSYCHOLOGICAL, EMOTIONAL

One emotion that certainly reaches our bones is fear and insecurity. Trembling is the powerful expression of fear governed by Bladder channel energies. Knowing how to balance fear with courage and wisdom is a refinement of the tasks the Bladder performs in body, heartmind, and spirit.

Sometimes courage can manifest as being pushy or possessing vaunting ambition. Both are expressions of yang Water energy. Mighty and inexorable, yang Water is a force that can carve canyons in the earth and forcefully make its way through human affairs.

Concomitant with this pushy ambitiousness can arise nervous anxiety. Factors could tip you off to the idea that you may have gone too far, pushed a little too hard, reached beyond your grasp just a bit too much, leaving you waiting for the other shoe to drop as a result.

Simply conjure the image of any maniacal leader in history who overextended his grasp of territory and resources, and you get a picture of how Bladder energy can lead to a rather dramatic collapse.

We are next led to the land of the deep unconscious, Water's province. In its yang aspect we will find the Bladder energy in governance in its more yin aspect we find the Kidney in charge.

Since the unconscious is by its nature a deep yin aspect of our essence, the influence related to Bladder energy will also be related to the effort that brings deep inner resources to the surface. Instinctual actions fall into this realm, those times when conditions in life can bring forth a primal response that surges from deep within.

And more often than not, these primal responses don't just come out of nowhere—there's actually a deep, programmed history involved. In many cases it is quite personal, having to do with your own personal life journey from zygote to fetus in the womb to infant, child, young adult, adult, senior, and ultimately freedom from the body through death.

This history of your life is like the flow of water. In fact, the Cherokee referred to water as "the long human being," equating humanity's long history with waters that flow on and on. The Bladder channel is thus the living existence of that long story in your body.

SPIRITUAL

The foundation for the spiritual levels of Bladder channel functions is the ultimate enactment of deep drives and instinctual, primal responses to the world within, through, and around you. The Bladder represents your connection and participation in the great ocean of life itself.

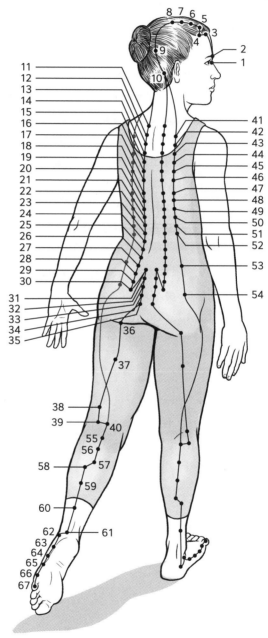

Figure 9: Bladder Meridian—Foot Tai Yang.

1. Bright Eyes
2. Silk Bamboo Bone
3. Eyebrow's Pouring
4. Crooked Curve
5. Fifth Palace
6. Receiving Light
7. Heavenly Connection
8. Declining Connection
9. Jade Pillow
10. Celestial Pillar
11. Great Shuttle
12. Wind Gate
13. Lung Transporter
14. Pericardium Transporter
15. Heart Transporter
16. Governor Transporter
17. Diaphragm Transporter
18. Liver Transporter
19. Gall Bladder Transporter
20. Spleen Transporter
21. Stomach Transporter
22. Triple Warmer Transporter
23. Kidney Transporter (Vitality Gate)
24. Sea of Qi Transporter
25. Large Intestine Transporter
26. Origin Gate Transporter
27. Small Intestine Transporter
28. Bladder Transporter
29. Mid Spine Transporter
30. White Ring Transporter
31. Upper Crevice
32. Second Crevice
33. Middle Crevice
34. Lower Crevice
35. Meeting of Yang
36. Brings Relief
37. Gate of Abundance
38. Floating Cleft
39. Outside the Crook
40. Middle of the Crook
41. Attached Branch
42. Door of the Corporeal Soul
43. Vital Region Transporter
44. Hall of the Spirit
45. Yi Xi
46. Diaphragm Gate
47. Gate of the Ethereal Soul
48. Yang's Key Link
49. Abode of Consciousness
50. Stomach Granary
51. Vitals Games
52. Residence of the Will
53. Bladder's Vitals
54. Order's Limit
55. Confluence of Yang
56. Support the Sinews
57. In the Mountains
58. Flying Yang
59. Instep Yang
60. Kunlun Mountains
61. Servant's Respect
62. Extending Vessel
63. Golden Gate
64. Captial Bone
65. Restraining Bone
66. Foot Connecting Valley
67. Extreme Yin

The Bladder Channel Trajectory

Inside the orbital ridge of the eye socket close to the bridge of the nose, the one meridian surfaces as the Bladder energy flow. Bladder 1, Bright Eyes, can be squeezed with thumb and forefinger each on opposite sides of the nose. With your eyes closed, this squeezing will generally create a bright light sensation, giving this point its name. Consider also our reflexive sensitivity to bright light; this point illustrates the interconnection of our eyes with the nervous system governed by the energy of Bladder channel and its partner, Kidney. This point is also the beginning point of the qiao mai, extraordinary vessel, the vessel of our stance. This vessel has much to do with our ability to be present in the here and now. Using our sense of vision and what we see is a powerful tool for maintaining presence.

From Bright Eyes, the Bladder energy takes its course up the forehead and over the top of the head, running in two parallel lines about an inch off centerline. At the base of the skull at the occipital ridge, clearly palpable where the upper trapezius muscle meets the occipital plate of the cranium, is Bladder 10, Celestial Pillar. We can see that the muscles of the back of the neck supporting the skull could be seen as pillars, given the concept of heaven above (the head), earth below.

From the Celestial Pillar, the Bladder meridian splits into two channels on each side, sending four channels of qi flowing down the back of the neck and the back of the body. These channels are referred to as the inner and outer branches of the Bladder meridian. We find Bladder 11 at the top of the back on the inner branch, which travels the more medial path all the way down the spine to the coccyx and continues down the thigh to the back of the knee to Bladder 40, Middle of the Crook. The outer branch starts at point number 41, Attached Branch, which is just lateral to Bladder 12 and streams the more lateral path down the back until it rejoins the inner branch at the back of the knee.

As we consider more deeply the significance of the location of this first section of the Bladder Meridian from 1 to 10 and 11, it is important to consider the relationship between the eyes, the base of the skull, and the neck. On the surface is a muscular relationship between the frontalis and the occipitalis muscles connected to one another by the broad tendonous sheath, the cranial aponeurosis, covering the skull. The occipitalis is in direct relationship with the all the muscles of the neck supporting the head and its rotational ability at the top the body. Deeper still are the eyes that connect to the visual cortex (located at the base of the skull) and the spinal column that begins at the back of the neck and carries the central nervous system from the brain all the way down the spinal cord to the base of the back. Together the muscles of the head, neck, and back can be considered at the service of the eyes and the entire nervous system, directing the sensory orifices found in the head up, down, back, front, and on either side. As we explore the Bladder meridian's range of functions, we will see again and again how closely connected it is to the necessity of orienting our head and its sensing organs—and indeed the entire body—to the environment surrounding us.

The channel splits into four lines, two on either side of the spine, and traverses the entire length of the back down to the tailbone. Consider how important it is to have a strong back and you'll discover a very important facet of the Bladder meridian's function. To have a strong Bladder channel is to have the ability to have a great capacity for meeting life's challenges.

Here in our back, the Bladder channel represents our unconscious and everything about ourselves we have difficulty looking at: it is our past and whatever motivates or pushes us from behind, providing much of the impetus necessary to move forward in the world.

How does motivation relate to the Bladder channel? It's simplistic, but consider the urge to urinate: a deep feeling that moves us from the inside, culminating in the realization that when you've got to go, you've got to go! On a more complex level, consider the many factors of family and culture that push us into the world, constraining us to behave within certain expected patterns. In classic literature, the Bladder channel is seen as the yang energy of the Water element manifesting in the body, and Water is related to our ancestors. Interestingly, the entire history of the genetic code of the human species is called the *gene pool*—not the "gene tree" or the "gene bonfire." And just as the power of Water is pervasive in our world, so too does its manifestation in our bodies speak of moving forward, sometimes slow and patient, sometimes fast and furious, but ever onward around that next obstacle toward whatever lies ahead.

From the top of the back to the bottom of the back, along the inner branch of the Bladder meridian are found a specific set of important points knows as the associated points, or transporter points. In Chinese these are called the *shu* points, in Japanese the *yu* points. Whatever language you use, the meaning is the same: these points relate to all channels of the body, and they both carry information about those channels and can be used to treat them. The function of carrying information for assessment and treatment is referred to as "transporting," and so these points are referred to as the transporting points. In other parts of this work you will find a complete list of these points, their locations, and their relationships. For this part in the discussion it is important to point out that every channel in the body can be accessed and treated through points found on the Bladder channel in the back, once more underlining its scope and importance.

From the tailbone and buttocks, the inner and outer branches of the Bladder channel continue down into the legs where they travel through the hamstrings to the back of the knee. The hamstring is an incredible muscle group that is potentially the strongest in the body (after the mandible) if we learn to develop and use it. These muscles propel the gymnast, martial artist, and ballerina through the air. When developed, a person can gain amazing strength and cover great distances. By the same token, weak hamstrings can cause the body myriad troubles, often a major culprit in back pain. A good Hatha yoga teacher will tell you that your back is hurting because your legs are weak. The muscles of the legs were designed to carry the weight of our bodies, the muscles of the back to stabilize us in an upright posture. If we attempt to use the back muscles to carry the weight of our bodies because our leg muscles are too weak to do it for us, our backs are vulnerable to injury and strain.

Finally reunited as one channel at the back of the knee, the Bladder proceeds from 40 down through the calves to Bladder 57, In the Mountains. This point rests right in the middle of the bifurcation of the gastrocnemius, or calf muscle. This powerful muscle facilitates jumping, climbing, running, and all activities of locomotion, and the point gets its name from the appearance of the muscle and its mountainous capacity to bear weight. Consider also hiking in mountainous terrain, as it places exquisite focus on this muscle and its relationship to the changing angles of the ankle when navigating uneven and sloping terrain.

From 57, the channel veers to the outside of the Achilles' tendon, passes behind the ankle bone and crosses to the foot, tracing the outer edge down to the final Bladder point at the baby toe, Bladder 67, Extreme Yin. A silly association that is nonetheless helpful in remembering the Bladder channel's completion at this humble point is the popular nursery rhyme in which "this little piggy cries wee, wee, wee, all the way home." Here the point name underscores an important principle of yin yang understanding, that when the energy of yang has run its course, it becomes yin. The next channel in the sequence, the Kidney channel, is referred to in the classics as Extreme Yin. We can see the energy of the Bladder meridian yielding its position to the next channel in the sequence, its yin partner in the Water element, the Kidney.

Kidney Meridian

Foot Shao Yin

The quality of Foot Shao Yin presents itself here in the body, beginning in the very bottom of the foot and rising up the back of the legs and thighs into the groin. This lesser yin quality is the most extreme yin, the deepest of the body.

Water Element

Representing the yin aspect of Water in the body, the Kidney channel holds the deep, essence of the human gene pool, our genetic lineage, and source of life in the body.

5 to 7 pm

This time of day comes after the afternoon lull, and we find a little perk of energy that carries us into the evening hours. This pick-me-up or second wind time of the day is attributed to the vitality of the kidney function.

Key Functions

Vitality, ancestral essence

Affirmation

I feel the vital life force flowing deep within me.

The Kidney channel of Foot Shao Yin is the yin representative of the Water element in the body. It charts a course from the bottom of the foot to the torso. It is known as the keeper of the ancestral energy and vitality of our being. On the physical level the kidneys purify the blood. A deep organ, their product is the fluid waste of all the bodily systems. Once they are done purifying the blood, they send it back to the lungs clean and ready for re-oxygenation. A main concept in Chinese medicine is that the Lungs bring in the qi or air, and the Kidneys reach up and grasp the qi from the lungs, pulling it down to light the fire of the Vitality Gate, the Ming Men Fire. The Ming Men Fire is the fire of life energy in the body.

The kidneys are known to govern vitality as it is closely related to the hormonal system, particularly the adrenal and corticoid glands. We can see their importance in the body's functioning dramatically if they should fail: the alternative is dialysis that must be performed daily. Most people in this situation suffer from an extreme sense of loss of vitality.

Another aspect of Kidney vitality as seen through Chinese medicine is its relationship to libido or sex drive. It is said that too much sex can damage the Kidneys, draining the vital essence. Good healthy Kidney function is further assessed through a healthy sex drive. More details of the Kidney function are drawn out in the descriptions that follow.

Key Characteristics of the Functional Range of the Kidney Channel
PHYSICAL
The Kidney channel governs the deepest aspects of our being and is found here in the most yin aspect of being, deep within. On a physical level it is related to the very purification of blood, the fluid of our vitality. Attached to that deep purification action is the Kidney channel function of hormone secretion and regulation as response to stressors.

The adrenal glands and cortisol production are under the direction and concern of the Kidney channel. The channel also governs our "get up and go" energy and fight or flight responses, our nervous system's interconnected sophisticated mechanisms of stimulus and response and the myriad synaptic feedback loops existing at every level of bodily organization.

And deep to this action of stimulus and response, fight or flight is the very felt sense of self-preservation in the face of danger and peril. In peaceful and quiet times, we turn to procreative activity, where the Kidney channel shows itself as governing the libido, the sexual drive, the procreative impulse—deeply rooted in a primal need to propagate.

Between the self-preservation instinct and the need to procreate is the ever-present task of balance. The inner ear is a fluid mechanism that reads the horizontal plane and keeps us right with it. In the face of all the twists and turns and rising and falling of life, the inner ear is our ship's keel. When the waters are stormy (or even when they are calm), the art of keeping balance as we shuttle through our world lands within the purview of Kidney channel functions.

In addition to being balanced via the inner ear's fluid mechanisms is the very sense of proprioception itself, that is, knowing where your body is in space at any given moment. From the bottoms of your feet to the tips of your fingers, from the tailbone to the crown, this whole body sensibility is the Kidney's realm of functioning.

Psychological, Emotional

What the physical level taught us about our physiology plays out in the psychological and emotional realms: cultivated patience, capacity, understanding, and wisdom. Fears and phobias that arise from the various life situations in which we find ourselves register here, and our response to them can lead to wising up or breaking down. The Kidney channel registers the full range of responses, and its depth of connection to our primal being grants us the capacity to meet the challenges of life and death.

Fight or flight responses are not just physical; they have strong psychological and emotional components as well. The literature on trauma documents thoroughly the often long-standing effects on the nervous system and attitude to life, learned behaviors that arise from the effects of intense experiences. All these intricate actions and reactions to the world around us can be attributed to the quality of Kidney energy.

Indeed, the ancestral energy flowing through us is an expression of these Kidney energies. The postures, positions, and dispositions that arise within us that are a direct reflection of what we inherited from our parents, grandparents, and great-grandparents as well as what we will pass on to our children, grandchildren, and great-grandchildren. This is the Kidney energy at work, the long view aspect of our humanity.

Classical Chinese texts break the Kidney function down into Kidney yin, Kidney yang, and Kidney qi. Kidney yin is the past, Kidney yang is the future, and Kidney qi is the present moment. From this, we can see the relationship of time to our human existence. Healthy Kidney channel energy will help us to balance our experiences of the past with our hopes for the future as we live fully in the present moment.

There is little denying that our personal relationship to the passage of time is often deeply wrapped up in our sense of family. Our parents, grandparents, siblings, and children all play a large part in the way we perceive time. As a result, any family-related stress we have can thus impact directly on our Kidney function. Maintaining poise, balance, and flow within family dynamics can be challenging in itself. As I look in the mirror of my family patterns, I ultimately come to see myself more clearly.

The actions of self-knowing, self-realization, and self-discovery are also Kidney channel functions. Here we find the Kidney closely connected to the Heart. As the Heart is governor of your truth and all you hold dear, the Kidney lies beneath it, supporting from below as it were. To get a sense of what that feels like, look to the nature of Fire and Water.

Fire is by its nature bright and warm, bringing things to the light. Water is dark, mysterious, and deep. One could think of Fire as consciousness and all that can be seen, and Water as the great unconscious—whatever is deep, reflective, and beneath the surface. Fire shows us the 10 percent tip of the iceberg, and Water represents the other 90 percent below the surface. Heart as Fire represents everything of which you are conscious and whatever you know about yourself, and Kidney as Water is all those things you have yet to learn about yourself that reveal themselves slowly over time and through experience. A favorite quote of mine that comes from the great Anonymous is "The road to truth is under construction." In other words, as much as we may know and be conscious of the present moment, there is always another layer waiting to be revealed.

It's no small wonder that fears and uncertainty can express themselves through deep and inward Kidney energy; it can often manifest in our lives as introversion and isolation.

Spiritual

Here we find ourselves at last at the spiritual manifestations and gifts of the Kidney channel, taking us to root-level issues of security, stability, and our sense of place and belonging in the world. Who we are as a people and how we survive being the fittest or most capable of collaboration—the deep intelligence necessary for our very survival itself—is governed by Kidney channel energy.

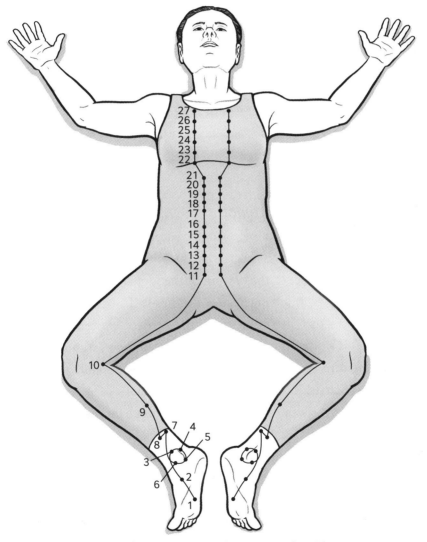

Figure 10: Kidney Meridian—Foot Shao Yin.

1. Bubbling Sping	15. Middle Flow
2. Blazing Valley	16. Vitals Transporter
3. Supreme Stream	17. Trade Winds Bend
4. Great Bell	18. Stone Pass
5. Water Spring	19. Yin Metropolis
6. Shining Sea	20. Abdomen Connecting Valley
7. Returning Current	21. Mysterious Gate
8. Exchange Belief	22. Walking Corridor
9. Guest House	23. Spirit Seal
10. Yin Valley	24. Spirit Ruin
11. Pubic Bone	25. Spirit Storehouse
12. Great Luminance	26. Comfortable Chest
13. Qi Cave	27. Transporter (Elegant) Mansion
14. Fourfold Fullness	

The Kidney Channel Trajectory

Kidney, the extreme yin channel, takes the baton and begins its turn along the course of the energy matrix. From the pinky toe, the one meridian goes inside to resurface at the bottom of the foot at an auspicious point known as Kidney 1, Bubbling Spring, just inside the edges of the ball of the foot. It is said that the yin energies of the earth enter the body through this point. It is a point that inspires a deep breath upon stimulation and has been used to revive the unconscious and lend support to those in emotional catharsis.

From here the Kidney energy travels up through the instep to the area behind and below the inner ankle bone. It makes a nice circle around and through this area, and those under stress will find pressure applied to these points to be quite sensitive and yet deeply stress reducing. From just behind the inner ankle the meridian moves up through the meeting point of the three yin leg meridians, Spleen 6, discussed prior, and then it travels up the inner aspect of the calf toward the back of the leg. It crosses through the tendons of the medial hamstrings at the inside back of the knee. From there it follows a course deep in the back of the thigh up to the medial border of the ischial tuberosity or sit bones. From the ischial tuberosity it traverses along the ischial and pubic rami to emerge right atop the pubic symphysis, Kidney 11, Pubic Bone, in the front of the body just a half-inch off centerline.

This trajectory through our "private zone" illustrates the Kidney channel's relationship to our innermost thoughts and feelings of life and death and our truly deep and vulnerable aspects. This area stretches mightily when in a squatting position, and for a woman in labor, dropping into a squatting position—the indigenous birthing position—calls forth a deep strength, as every woman who has delivered this way can attest. In this archetypal posture we can clearly see the great power of the Kidney function in the regulation of hormones and vitality and the preservation of ancestral essence.

From the pubic area the channel continues just a half-inch off the centerline, rising through the abdomen to the solar plexus. The points 12, Great Luminence; 13, Qi Cave; 14, Fourfold Fullness; 15, Middle Flow; 16, Vitals Transporter; 17, Trade Winds Bend; 18, Stone Pass; 19, Yin Metropolis; and 20, Abdomen Connecting Valley all evoke the auspiciousness of this channel and its action in the body. At the solar plexus, the channel enters the rib cage at Kidney 21, Mysterious Gate, a point where the great qi of the abdomen flows into the great qi of the chest to nourish that most myterious of organs, the heart. The channel then widens out into the chest to about two inches from centerline with points between each rib. From 22, Walking Corridor; 23, Spirit Seal; 24, Spirit Ruin; 25, Spirit Storehouse; and 26, Comfortable Chest, we find a set of points directly related to ancestral or spirit energy.

The abdomenal and thoracic points of the Kidney and their evocotive names truly illuminate this energy channel's deep and powerful nature. Our own colloquial expressions in English such as "playing your cards close to your chest" or "getting something off your chest" are phrases that resonate with the functioning of this important channel. Through stimulation of this area, anything you are holding on to, or that is holding on to you at this level can be released and transformed.

The Kidney energy channel comes to an end just under the inner corner of the collar bone. Kidney 27, Transporter Mansion or Elegant Mansion, is the last stop on the Kidney line. Like the transporting points of the Bladder meridian, Kidney 27 is the transport point of all the transport points. Here the entire energy system of the body can be assessed and treated. Also known as the adrenal pump, stimulation of this point activates the vital energy of the body, heartmind, and spirit.

Chapter 6

Protection and Circulation

In this chapter we explore the Pericardium and Triple Warmer channels of qi and their functions in body, heartmind, and spirit. Note that these lines constitute the Jue Yin and Shao Yang aspects of the supplemental Fire force. They are located in the body along the sides of the arms.

Pericardium Meridian

Hand Jue Yin

The Pericardium channel correlates to the muscle of the heart. As it surrounds the heart, it is not as "deep" as the heart itself. Where the Heart holds the space of Shao Yin (deepest yin), Pericardium holds the space of Jue Yin, middle yin. And we see this also in relation to the Lung, the Tai Yin (greater yin) or most superficial of the yin organs. The Lung is indeed on the surface, interfacing directly with incoming air. The Pericardium is deeper in the body than this, though not as deep as the Heart. And so we find Jue Yin, middle yin, as the energy quality of the Pericardium function. The channel itself runs a course from the torso, out the arm, to the third finger.

Supplemental Fire Element

Supplemental Fire is a conceptualization of a secondary aspect of the Fire element as it expresses itself in the human form. If absolute Fire is equated to the attribute of being warm-blooded (an optimal body temperature of 37º C/98.6º F), then supplemental Fire is the warm coat we wear to keep that body temperature regulated when the thermometer outside drops below freezing. Supplemental Fire is the "extra" fire we need to keep the inner fire protected and burning brightly. It is not a principle that plays out only with clothing; it also plays out in our diets, housing, and a social environment that supports warm and loving human connections.

7 to 9 pm

This time of day is often considered the most social: "Dinner at 8 and don't be late." Traditionally at this time the day's work has been finished, and we gather around the hearth to share stories, comfort, food, sustenance, libations, and simply human care.

Key Functions

Circulation, emotions

Affirmation

I open my heart with compassion for all life has to offer.

The Pericardium channel of Hand Jue Yin is the yin channel of the supplemental Fire in the body, heartmind, and spirit. As was said above like its yang partner, Triple Warmer, it is not named after an organ western anatomical science has identified, and this aspect of these channels teaches us much about what meridian systems are. Consider the body as wrapped in an energic exoskeleton, the channel system's energy matrix.

Roughly parallel to the body's musculo-skeletal, circulatory, and nervous, channels of qi are considered the governing system over all these physical functions. The qi in the channels and throughout body tissues harmonizes and coordinates all the parts of the body, heartmind, and spirit, linking and connecting, while simultaneously fueling and inspiring the system in its daily and seasonal cycles.

The energy of life is one single force. It passes throughout the body, heartmind, and spirit, taking on all the various tasks of life on its journey. One cannot truly look at the system as separate functioning systems unless this singular life energy concept and all its interactive aspects is taken into account.

One action does not happen independent of any other. One action comes from the whole and goes back to the whole, moving the organism forward, backward, upward, downward, and from side to side.

The energy of life is not constrained to the functioning of physical organs alone but rather to the overall functioning of life on all levels—physical, mental, emotional, and spiritual. To this end, the Pericardium and Triple Warmer channels assist us in making the leap of awareness from physical organ function to the comprehensive, holistic functioning of qi energy.

Truly the energy of life itself flows throughout the body, heartmind, and spirit as long as we are alive. An autopsy will not yield evidence of meridian pathways or channels of living qi, for once the physical vessel has passed from life to death, life energy leaves behind no traces.

The key functions of the Pericardium channel are related to circulation and emotionality. It is said to be the chief minister in charge of the defense of the Heart. If all the buffets and blows of life were directly impact the heart, it would fail much sooner. A healthy Pericardium, on the other hand, can absorb the shocks and keep the heart protected. The effects of emotional trauma, crimes of passion, mood, and affect are all related to and governed by the quality of the Pericardium channel's energy.

Key Characteristics of the Functional Range of the Pericardium Channel

PHYSICAL

The Pericardium is responsible for the health of blood vessels. Blood pressure, high or low, can be attributed to and treated through the Pericardium system.

Pericardial tissue is the muscle that surrounds the heart. Its health is vital to the overall function of circulation throughout the body.

PSYCHOLOGICAL, EMOTIONAL

As the muscle tissue surrounding the heart, we can see that the pericardium exists in service to the heart itself and its protection. It is charged with the noble duty as the first line of contact with the world around us, and it keeps an eye on that contact to ensure it is safe for the Heart and us.

This place—emotions, feelings, our moods, and all affect—is the realm of the Pericardium. It relates to our ability to "read" or "check the temperature" of an emotional environment, critical to our survival and protection.

It can be seen from this that the nature and quality of our human relationships is central to the Pericardium's function. The give and take of love, care, and concern are central to this vital function. Many sentimental song lyrics immortalize this aspect of human life.

The notions of sentimentality and love are related to the emotional aspects of sexual experience. It's not just the physical sexual drive at stake here. That is the realm of the Kidney and the procreative function.

Here we are speaking of the feelings of love themselves; care, concern, shared warmth, affection, vulnerability, sensitivity, spontaneity of loving expression, and excitement or the lack of any of these human aspects of lovemaking are at the core of the Pericardium's service in our lives.

SPIRITUAL

At the highest level, the spiritual teaching of Pericardium is that love is the answer. And the virtues of kindness and care and safe holding of all that is precious is the spiritual imperative of the Pericardium function.

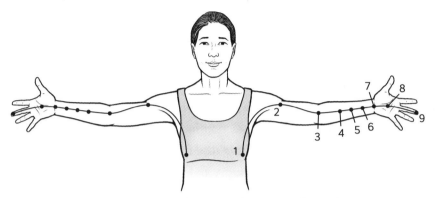

Figure 11: Pericardium Meridian—Hand Jue Yin.

1. Heaven's Pond
2. Heavenly Spring
3. Marsh at the Crook
4. Xi-Cleft Gate
5. Intermediate Messenger

6. Inner Frontier Gate
7. Great Mound
8. Palace of Toil
9. Central Rushing

Trajectory of the Pericardium Channel

From Kidney 27 our one meridian once again drops into the inner body to travel to a point just an inch lateral to the nipple. Here the energy of the Pericardium channel emerges. Spoken of as the energy that protects the Heart from the buffets and blows of life, the location of this channel speaks for itself. Its very first point Pericardium 1, Heaven's Pond, refers with great reverence to the reservoir of breast milk that nourishes humans in infancy and early childhood. One has but to notice the beatific contentment on the face of a child just after nursing to grasp the significance of this name. And in this simple act, the infant is being reassured that it is safe, loved, and well cared for as it begins its journey in this strange land of life.

From the breast, the Pericardium channel rises through the pectorals and out into the arm. It courses through the trough-like structure between the two muscle bundles from which the biceps derive their name. It then passes through the inner crease of the elbow and through the center of the forearm on a pathway parallel to and in between the ulna and radius. Three fingers before it reaches the wrist lies Pericardium 6, Inner Frontier Gate, a point known to cure motion sickness and to help smokers to kick the habit. As the Inner Gate, it also has much to do with introspection and one's relationship with oneself. Much protection for the Heart can be derived from knowing oneself. Great danger lies ahead for those who are unaware on an internal level of their own true nature and preciousness.

Crossing the wrist fold, the Pericardium channel rests at the center of the palm at Pericardium 8, Palace of Toil. The image of toiling in the fields, at the office, or at home to provide for the family or the village is reflected in the hardworking hands. Likewise, to grasp and caress are actions of the hand that reflect the function of the Pericardium opening and closing in like measure, like the muscle of the heart. A psychologist working with a group of hardened alcoholics captured this image perfectly: "You've all learned to do this really well," he said, making a fist. "Now all you have to do, is learn to do this," and he opened his palm, holding out his hand in an offer of service. Alternately known as the Palace of Anxiety, Pericardium 8 is the site of our nervous hand wringing and sweating. To soothe stage fright and jitters, we rub this spot.

Finally, the meridian comes to a close at the pad at the end of the middle finger, Pericardium 9, Central Rushing. The strongest and longest finger of the hand, it was known in the ancient world as the finger of wisdom. Indeed, it takes great wisdom to know the courage of the Heart and live by it, just as it is important to surround yourself with others who care about you and would stand by you through good times and bad. Here at the tip of the middle finger, the yin energies of the Pericardium represent the farthest reach of the hand. We recognize here the yin reaching the yang, just as the yang reached the yin at Bladder 67.

Triple Warmer Meridian

Hand Shao Yang

The Shao Yang quality is called the "lesser yang," "weakest yang," or "younger yang." If Tai Yang of Small Intestine is the greatest, and Yang Ming of Large Intestine is the sunlight, then here we find Shao Yang as the slightest of the yang factors. Shao Yang resides in the side of the body, the most lateral aspect of our being. To illustrate, consider the following "courtroom" or legal drama that plays out in the arms. There are three characters in any courtroom procedural drama: the prosecuting attorney, the defense attorney, and the judge/jury. The Large Intestine, Hand Yang Ming, expressing itself through the pointer finger is our prosecuting attorney. The Small Intestine, the Hand Tai Yang, is the judge/jury expressing through the pinky finger and the falling of the gavel that calls for order in the courtroom and reads out the sentence. And the Triple Warmer, Hand Shao Yang, is the defense attorney, flowing expressively through the fourth finger, the back of the hand the outside of the wrist, used for blocking the oncoming blows in any bout.

Supplemental Fire Element

As we explored the supplemental Fire and its relationship to absolute Fire above, the same applies here with Triple Warmer. The gradation to consider here is that this is the yang expression of supplemental Fire. Where Pericardium governs the yin expression and the inward focus of protection and emotions and concerns for the heart's continued beating, the yang aspect refers more to protections from external influences, and we find the Triple Warmer deeply involved in all manner of immune response. The safety of the body, heartmind, and spirit as a whole from the smallest invasion of bacteria in a minor cut to the invasion of tumorous, cancerous growths is where Triple Warmer is called to action.

9 to 11 pm

This exquisite time of day is the time when Triple Warmer runs highest. At night clubs, things are just beginning to warm up. On television, the more "adult programming" begins. In the bedroom, the wise are retiring and snuggling under the comforter.

Key Functions

Immune system, protective mechanisms

Affirmation

I protect the precious life that is given to me.

The Triple Warmer channel of Hand Shao Yang is the yang aspect of supplemental Fire in the body, heartmind, and spirit. It has no physical organ correlative, thus giving us insight into the nature of the energetic channel system. Its range of functions is wide. Known as the Great Regulator channel, it is in charge of regulating body temperature and the smooth communication of energy throughout the being, smoothly disseminating qi throughout the entire network of meridian functions. A primary focus of its functionality can be seen in its relationship to protection. Triple Warmer provides a line of defense as it maintains an even temperature throughout the system. The name itself is derived from the understanding of the three burning spaces, the upper, middle, and lower aspects of the body that correlate to circulation and respiration, digestion and assimilation, and reproduction and elimination. Triple Warmer is charged with the duty of making sure an optimal temperature is maintained for all of these functions. An understanding of Triple Warmer's role can be seen when studying its elemental nature. As the yang aspect of supplemental Fire, the emphasis is not on core fire but rather the mechanisms that protect it; it's extra fire we need to maintain our core fire. In winter it is a warm blanket, a fireplace, an overcoat; in summer it is a cool dip in the lake, cooling foods and beverages, bug repellant, sunscreen, and mosquito netting.

Triple Warmer also relates to the people with whom we surround ourselves to provide the support we need to live full, healthy, and satisfying lives. Important self-protection is derived from our significant personal relationships.

Masunaga in *Zen Shiatsu* beautifully describes these critical interpersonal aspects of Triple Warmer function, giving a brilliant snapshot of its role in social relationships, preparedness, and protection when he speaks of being "overprotected as a child, thrown out into the world unprepared," a definitive symptom of deficient qi in the Triple Warmer. More details about its functional range can be found in the descriptions that follow.

Key Characteristics of the Functional Range of the Triple Warmer Channel

PHYSICAL

On the physical level, Triple Warmer governs and regulates body temperature taking care to maintain 37°C/98.6°F throughout the body. When in the presence of foreign invaders, it will invoke a fever to drive out the invasion. A clear expression of this immune response, the lymphatic system and all the T-cells designed to fight off pathogenic invasion are related to the Triple Warmer.

PSYCHOLOGICAL, EMOTIONAL

When we take the physical into the psychological realm, we are bound to explore the entire range of interpersonal interaction. Of main concern in our psychological environment is our relationship with our social group, beginning with our family of origin, our parents, and the culture in which we are raised.

It is generally our primary caregivers who first teach us the prescribed way of dealing with the world and its conditions. They button up our coats, pull on our boots, and otherwise teach us how to be prepared and ready for the outside world. Any issues we have or have had with our parents resonate here in the Triple Warmer, where the ways in which we protect ourselves emotionally and interpersonally are all interwoven.

Whether we are friendly, personable, and gregarious, or distant, introverted, and isolated all correlate to this function. In short, all the psycho-emotional components of life are reflected in this channel.

SPIRITUAL

At the spiritual level, Triple Warmer speaks to our longing for connection; indeed, it is our very sense of love and belonging.

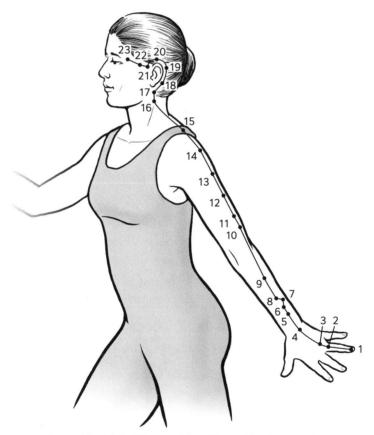

Figure 12: Triple Warmer Meridian—Hand Shao Yang.

1. Rushing Pass
2. Fluid Gate
3. Central Islet
4. Yang Pool
5. Outer Frontier Gate
6. Branch Ditch
7. Ancestral Meeting
8. Three Yang Meeting
9. Four Rivers
10. Heavenly Will
11. Clear Cold Abyss
12. Dispersing River
13. Upper Arm Meeting
14. Shoulder Crevice
15. Heavenly Crevice
16. Window of Heaven
17. Wind Screen
18. Spasm Vessel
19. Skull's Rest
20. Minute Angle
21. Ear Gate
22. Ear Harmony Crevice
23. Silk Bamboo Hollow

Triple Warmer Channel Trajectory

The powerful middle finger represents the terminus point for Pericardium energies; the one meridian goes inward once again to reemerge at the tip of the fourth, or ring finger, where the Triple Warmer energies rise to the surface. Triple Warmer governs the functions of shared warmth, protection, and overall distribution and regulation of life energy. Just as with the Pericardium, there is no direct physical organ correlate to the Triple Warmer, rather it provides an overall regulatory function for the entire system. The "triple" in its name refers to the Chinese understanding of the division of the body, heartmind, and spirit into three burning spaces: upper, middle, and lower. The upper burner encompasses intellectuality, respiration, and circulation. The middle burner governs digestion and assimilation. The lower burner supplies the necessary warmth for elimination and reproduction. The image of a burner or a warmer refers to the fact that we are warm-blooded creatures and as such, temperature regulation is critical in the maintenance of our optimal functioning. Reading your overall body temperature is fundamental to health assessment. Triple Warmer is the channel system directly responsible for maintaining our thermal nature.

As to the functional aspects of the Triple Warmer that help us to grasp an understanding of why the surface trajectory is located where it is, we need to focus on the understanding of protection and shared warmth. As the meridian begins its surface manifestation, we are struck by its location on the fourth finger, the ring finger. This finger symbolizes marriage, bonding for life in pledge of mutual support and sharing. And our marriage is the place where ideally we create the protective home life through relationship, partnership, and shared warmth. Our marital partner knows us most intimately and can provide for us a safe haven and a place where we can be ourselves. It is of course interesting to note that at the same time that we are most protected here, it is also the place where we are most vulnerable, an aspect of yin and yang that is most revealing. If we were not vulnerable there would be nothing to protect, and yet through sharing that vulnerability within the safe ring of a marital confidant, we actually increase our sense of protection.

This Triple Warmer protective quality continues on through the back of the hand to the backhand of the forearm. This area is used for blocking punches in martial arts practice, and in the sport of tennis it provides a powerful swing angle that preserve's a player's ability to remain in the volley. Four fingers proximal to the wrist fold we find Triple Warmer 5, the Outer Frontier Gate. This is directly opposite Pericardium 6, Inner Frontier Gate. As the Inner Gate has to do with introversion, conversely the Outer Gate has to do with extroversion. With the yin meridian, we look inward, with the yang meridian we face outward. How do we face the world that surrounds us, interfacing with it and also protecting ourselves from the world's more threatening aspects? The alternate name Flying Tiger is given to this point, a reference to the mythical beast who, when your ally, becomes a strong protective force for you. A tiger is of course dangerous enough on land; when it is flying, you want to make sure it is on your side! During World War II, a US Air Force squadron stationed in mainland China to defend against the Japanese invasion was named the Flying Tigers to evoke public confidence in the Allied efforts. This strong name is also given to this auspicious point located on the Triple Warmer on the back of the forearm, demonstrating this strong aspect of our being, seen as the front line of our defense against the buffets and blows of life.

Another way to see the relationship between the channel's location and its function is to notice that this it is found on the "sunny side" of the arm. This side of the arm catches the most sun, and manifests our suntan, sunburn, and freckles. It's literally the aspect of our body which takes the heat.

Over the back corner of the elbow, the Triple Warmer passes through 10, Heavenly Will, and then passes up through the triceps. This is the area of the arm where you rub warmth back into yourself on a chilly evening. Or you may find yourself wrapping your arms around another as they wrap theirs around you to keep warm and snug. On that same evening, you may find your shoulders rising to your ears to protect your neck and ears from the cold. The large muscles of the upper trapezius are responsible for this action, and the Triple Warmer passes right through the middle of this muscle.

The channel continues up into the sides of the neck to meet the skull just under the ear, and then tracks around behind the ear at the hairline. The names of 17, Wind Screen, and 19, Skull Rest, really capture the quality of the energy behind the ear. It then circles around to the "sideburns" and cuts across the temples to its final point 23, Silk Bamboo Hollow, just off the end of the eyebrow. The image of laying your head upon your pillow and snuggling up beneath the comforter directly evokes both the location and the function of the Triple Warmer energy channel. A gentle circular rubbing or stroking of the temple at 23 will soothe your overworked, stressed out mind.

Chapter 7

Sense of Direction

In this chapter we explore the Gall Bladder and Liver channels of qi and their functions in body, heartmind, and spirit. These lines constitute the Jue Yin and Shao Yang aspects of the Wood elemental force and are located in the body along the sides of the legs.

Gall Bladder Meridian

Foot Shao Yang

Just as Triple Warmer shows us the expression of Shao Yang in the arms, the Gall Bladder shows us the Shao Yang in the legs. The Gall Bladder here is explained in relation to the Stomach and the Bladder: the Stomach represents the yang ming, reflecting all those motivations that pull us forward into life (the proverbial carrot dangling in front of us), and the Bladder represents the Tai Yang, governing all those motivations of drive, pushing from deep within, or escaping whatever is chasing us. For its part, the Gall Bladder represents the Shao Yang, giving us the possibility to move from side to side and the choice to go right or left.

We may wonder: how does Shao Yang show us the lesser yang? Here I like to say that an enticing carrot in front of you or a big bear chasing you are very straightforward and powerful motivations. But the decision to turn right or left is always subject to scrutiny. Deciding to turn right, I may be tempted to question my choice or defend it, and these are two very weak positions.

Wood Element

And here we find the Wood element expressing itself in the body. In the five element system of Chinese medicine are Fire, Earth, Metal, Water, and Wood. Anyone schooled in the Western four-element system is familiar with Fire, Earth, Air, and Water and may ask, "Where is Air in the Chinese system?" It's a curious task to compare two ways of looking at nature and its expressions. Western Air is most closely correlated to the Chinese Metal element, yet we may also see some Air-like characteristics appearing in Wood. Indeed, an alternative name for Wood is Wind. It is not my intention nor within the scope of this book to do a full comparison of various cultures' systems of natural perception; suffice it to say that Wood captures the natural quality of a force that is persistent, strong, deeply rooted, and organic. It grows from the soils of earth, nourished or inhibited by its minerals and metals and likewise the waters that run over and through it; it is both inspired to growth by the power of fire as the sun calling it forth and can also be used as fuel for our fires. Wood is the vital element of organic growth and all the powers granted or inhibited by such growth.

11 pm to 1 am

The Gall Bladder channel spans the hours of 11 pm to 1 am, the night owl's energies. These are the hours when sensible people are in bed, at rest and sleeping after a long day. And for those who are young and restless, these can be the hours when the night is young and mischief is afoot. Parties come to life and all manner of nighttime shenanigans commence at this hour. If you are up and partying at this hour and find yourself with a case of the midnight munchies, it's likely you will not reach for a salad or smoothie—more likely it will be pizza, ice cream, or some greasy and salty snack. Because the Gall Bladder concentrates bile—a strong emulsifier or grease cutter—it is really put to the test by any fatty foods consumed at this hour! You may also notice the two-hour cycle manifesting strongly here. Many people will agree that if you are not asleep by 11, you'll be up until 1.

Key Functions
Decision making, distribution center

Affirmation
I stand my ground with strength and integrity.

The Gall Bladder channel of Foot Shao Yang is the yang channel of the Wood element that runs along the lateral aspect of the body from the head to the feet. It is the yang aspect of the Wood element in the human body, heartmind, and spirit. On the physical level it governs the distribution of nutrients throughout the body; on the mental and emotional levels it animates responsibility and decision-making. Named after the gall bladder organ, the organ itself is known to concentrate and store bile produced by the liver and then excrete it into the small intestine upon demand. Bile is an emulsifier, a substance that breaks down fat (fuel). The gall bladder is an essential player in the breaking down of fats into constituent parts so they may be assimilated into the bloodstream and sent to the liver for further processing into nutrients for cell functioning throughout the body. We see Gall Bladder as the assistant to the Liver and vital in the work of supplying nutrients.

When we go beyond this physical level of functioning, we consider the word "gall" itself to help us come to an understanding of this channel's characteristic, To say one has a lot of gall speaks to a sense of nerve and belligerence. Someone with a lot of gall gets things done despite the odds or at least will go down swinging. Someone with a strong Gall Bladder function may have a reputation as a reliable or hard worker and a good decision-maker who can be counted on to stick with it through thick and thin. These sorts of people are good sidekicks. While not usually "idea people," they might come up with good strategies. Overall vision is more the domain of the chief executive—in this case the Liver channel—whose functions we explore below.

Key Characteristics of the Functional Range of the Gall Bladder Channel

PHYSICAL

The physical gall bladder serves the physical function of concentrating and secreting bile in to the duodenum, the first section of the Small Intestine. As mentioned above, bile is a strong emulsifier, it breaks down fats into constituent parts so the small intestine can better glean nutrients from dietary fats and oils. In addition to being an emulsifier, bile is also a strong alkaline substance. After the strong acidic environment of the stomach, a strong alkaline influence must be exerted to bring the digesta (the liquid slurry of food created through mastication and the action of the stomach) into a balanced pH for moving through the small intestine. Without the alkalinization process, stomach acid would burn the small intestine's lining and cause gastric ulcers.

Beyond these functions, the Gall Bladder channel energy has a broader physical function in being involved with the actual distribution of nutrients throughout body. Generally considered to be a function of blood, the distinction here is less about the actual medium that carries the nutrient and more about the allotment and even distribution of the right nutrients to the right cells and tissues at the right times.

In this regard, the Gall Bladder channel is also in charge of the body's muscular action. Consider the muscles' action as being an organic function of movement, growth, and choice. Like the characteristics of Wood explored earlier, you can see the muscles as the manifestation of the living quality of Wood in the body. Healthy muscles are flexible and pliable like young willow branches. Diseased muscles are stiff and rigid like an old oak, or weak and flaccid like a leaf floating on a lake or smoke on the wind.

PSYCHOLOGICAL, EMOTIONAL

The physical attributes of musculature and the digestive system have correlation in our psycho-emotional layer as the energy behind repetitive and even addictive behaviors. Our habits of body are correlated to our habits of mind. When we are busy doing, doing, doing we are like the many branches of a tree reaching out in all directions at once. And here you can also see the strength of the tree as being exemplary of being reliable and responsible. Gall Bladder energy governs the virtues of dependability and integrity.

Call to mind if you can what it might be like to own a luxurious yacht. You moor it in, say, Miami Beach or San Diego. Most of the year you live in some big northern city where you have an expensive, luxurious high-rise condo. I know this is not the norm for everyone, but imagine if you did own such a vessel in such a situation, you would know that you need to hire a capable and reliable first mate. Your luxury, high-rise condo already comes pre-staffed with a cadre of capable security and maintenance professionals. For your yacht, you'd have to hire your own first mate, someone who would live on the yacht and keep it in ship shape and ready to sail at a moment's notice. This person would have to be of high integrity, extremely responsible, capable, and ever ready for your command. At the same time, the person would need to treat your yacht as if it were their own. Such a highly responsible position is the exact definition of Gall Bladder energy. This vital energy channel governs anywhere in your life you rely on others to keep it all together for you and your dearest possessions, or where you do the same for others.

What goes hand in hand with such a high level of responsibility is the ability to be in control. And so all control issues show up as a feature of the Gall Bladder energy system. If you are in control, want to be in control, need to be in control, have to let go of control, aren't in control, or need to surrender control to a higher power, these are all aspects of your Gall Bladder's function. You may notice how these can all be directly related to anger. Consider the hair-trigger response some people can have when any aspect of control (or lack of it) is challenged, and you'll see how the two are directly related.

Anger is not limited to issues of control or lack thereof; it also relates to issues of creativity and the frustration of creative impulse. Anger is an essential primal reaction we have when things are not going right according to our sense of how things ought to be going. In this way, anger has a vitally important role in causing us to immediately figure out what is true for us. It can alert us to the fact that we are experiencing something uncomfortable related to a thing we care for very much. If we did not care, we would not get angry.

The right recognition of anger can clue us in as to what is most important. Of course, when anger runs amok, it can become senseless violence and rage, deeply related to the struggles of addiction, control, and obsession. These too are intertwined with the proper functioning of Gall Bladder energy within the body, heartmind, and spirit. Bullying and bossing come from the same place. A good boss guides employees in the successful accomplishment of an important task. A bully enforces power over others in a rude, inappropriate, and hateful fashion.

To face all these issues means to balance your relationship with power. You can be bold and courageous in the face of overwhelming odds and fight for a cause you believe in, or you can become pompous, self-important, and arrogant if the scale tips a little too much. There is often a fine line between power and right, and many a tyrant has run afoul the mantle of leadership. "Absolute power corrupts absolutely" is a warning against the misuse of Gall Bladder energy in social and political systems.

SPIRITUAL

The spiritual call of Gall Bladder Foot Shao Yang energy is growth, dedication, reliability, and good old-fashioned integrity. The wise admonition for conducting important interpersonal relations is the spiritual imperative of the Gall Bladder channel: say what you mean, mean what you say.

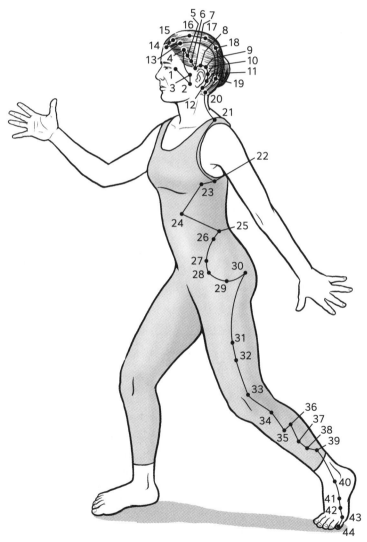

Figure 13: Gall Bladder Meridian—Foot Shao Yang.

1. Seeing the World
2. Meeting of Hearing
3. Above the Joint
4. Jaw Serenity
5. Wild Skull
6. Wild Tuft
7. Crook of the Temple
8. Leading Valley
9. Heavenly Rushing
10. Many Voices
11. Inner Listening
12. Getting Into Action
13. Root of the Spirit
14. Yang White (Third Eye Opening)
15. Head Overlooking Tears
16. Window of the Eyes (See the Face of God)
17. Upright Nourishment (God Sees You)
18. Supporting Spirit
19. Brain Hollow
20. Pond of Wind
21. Well in the Shoulder
22. Armpit Abyss
23. Flank Sinews
24. Sun and Moon
25. Capital Gate
26. Girdling Vessel
27. Five Pivots
28. Linking Path
29. Stationary Crevice
30. Jumping Pivot
31. Market of Wind
32. Middle Ditch
33. Knee Yang Gate
34. Yang Mound Spring
35. Yang Intersection
36. Outer Hill
37. Bright Light
38. Yang Assistance
39. Suspended Bell
40. Mound of Ruins
41. Foot Overlooking Tears
42. Earth Five Meetings
43. Clamped Stream
44. Foot Yin Portal

Gall Bladder Channel Trajectory

The temple region and behind the ear is the territory of the Triple Warmer, that area soothed by gentle, warm, circular stroking. Its location also manifests in the meridian flow. We recognize the Gall Bladder and the Triple Warmer as being expressions of the Shao Yang energy of the body's sides. Our one meridian goes inward after Triple Warmer 23 and travels a scant inch down to just outside the outer orbital ridge of the eye to the first point on the Gall Bladder channel in the area where crow's feet are known to form, 1, Seeing the World. From there the pathway flows down to the ear where two points manifest and then goes up into the curve of hair that rims the temples. Here there are four points running parallel to the hairline; one of them, GB 6, is called Wild Tuft, an apt description of the hair at the temples that often sticks out in a wild and crazy way. It is also related to the way a whirlwind of activity can lead to a kind of wild and crazy spinning that can really mess up your hairdo.

From the temple hairline, the channel flows back around the ear an inch inside the hairline. This is parallel to the Triple Warmer channel that flows on the hairline around the ear. It is valuable to self-palpate these two lines in order to distinguish their slightly different character. Closer to the ear on the hairline you get one feeling, and just an inch inside the hairline is quite a different feeling.

The Gall Bladder continues around the skull to GB 12, Getting Into Action, at the occipital ridge. It then tracks up to the forehead where it continues. GB 13, 14, and 15 make a triangle: 13 and 15 are just at the hairline and 14 is in the middle of the forehead in alignment with the eyes. From 15, Head Overlooking Tears, the channel traces a line back over the side of the head, following a course about two inches lateral of the midline.

When the line reaches the occipital ridge once more, we find Gall Bladder 20, Pond of Wind. This name evokes images related to Gall Bladder's role as decision-maker. With all of life's information swirling like the wind over a small pond, we must choose our way. In fact, the entire first section of the Gall Bladder—from its start just outside the eyes to the ears, to its trace along the sides of the head in two lines and its point directly above the eyes, as well as points 12 and 20 at the occipital ridge—we find the location directly relates to turning the head side to side; it is the ability to see both sides of a situation and make a decision to go right or left. This auspicious positioning in the sides of the head lends weight and reason to its role as the decision-maker, for as every school child learns, we must look both ways before crossing the road.

From 20, the pathway drops down the sides of the neck, crossing over the Triple Warmer channel as it makes its way to Gall Bladder 21, Well in the Shoulder. Here it sits deep in the tissue, midway between the clavicle and the scapula and midway from the corner of the shoulder to the base of the neck. This point relates to Gall Bladder's task of bearing responsibilities. Often when we are bearing burdens that are too great, we manifest pain or injury in the shoulder region. Gall Bladder 21 is the perfect point for assisting to relieve the tension in our shoulders that is the result of the bearing of our responsibilities, both real and assumed.

From 21, the Gall Bladder channel then goes around the front of the shoulder and through the pectorals toward two points in the fourth intercostal space just below the armpit. Then it travels forward to the seventh intercostal space to Gall Bladder 24, Sun and Moon, found at a point in line with the nipple. The name is significant to the point's use and effectiveness: sun and moon are yang and yin; though the meridian is yang, the Gall Bladder crosses to this yin area of the body, and stimulating it can bring balance to the yin and yang of the body. The point is also the "alarm point" for the Gall Bladder channel and is used to assess and treat acute conditions of the Gall Bladder.

After 24 the channel shifts toward the back again, to a point at the tip of the twelfth rib—25, Capital Gate. This point is the Kidney's alarm point. Bearing a special relationship to it and as the Capital Gate, this point is seen as an important point for accessing and treating the source qi.

From here the channel crosses forward once more, cross the waistline to trace the delicate area just anterior and medial to the anterior iliac crest. There are two points here, which when palpated might induce a tickle response, so one should be careful in stimulating this area. From here the channel traces down and back once more into the buttocks to Gall Bladder 30, Jumping Pivot, deep in the hip socket.

From Gall Bladder 21, the Well in the Shoulder, to 30, Jumping Pivot, we see the run of the Gall Bladder in the torso. It is a busy channel, running front to back many times. This is reflective of the channel's task as the distributor of qi to all the systems of the body. Its strong presence in the body's side also illustrates its task as decision-maker. It has influence on both sides of the body, a metaphor for the two sides of a situation. Seeing both sides is a necessity so that proper data can be gathered to make a good decisions, one of the Gall Bladder channel's key functions.

Finally, the Gall Bladder enters the legs and straightens its path right along the pants seam, tracing the iliotibial (IT) band in the thigh. Just a little past the halfway point between hips and knee we find Gall Bladder 31, Market of Wind. Another wind point, this name refers to Gall Bladder's connection with Wood that bears a close relationship to elemental Air or Wind. The "market" part of the name speaks to a level of decision-making one must do in situations like at a marketplace. To be successful, a merchant must be able to read the winds of public need and desire and find a position for properly catching that wind for optimal gain. As the strategist of the team of functions, the Gall Bladder is directly responsible for choosing positions.

The channel continues down the leg, crossing over the lateral side of the knee joint and over the head of the fibula. The fibula is known as the assistant bone in Western anatomy for the way in which it assists the tibia, the shinbone. We see here a mirror to the Chinese idea that the Gall Bladder is the assistant to the Liver. When we explore the Liver trajectory later, we will find that the Liver channel follows the tibia. The Gall Bladder traces a course along the assistant bone, perfectly illustrating its supportive nature. Just inferior to the head of the fibula lies GB 34, Yang Mound Spring. Its name is derived from its function as a spring point and its location on a yang meridian just under the "mound" of the head of the fibula. As a spring point it is considered a deep and pure source of yang qi. This auspicious point is said to have a strong influence over all the sinews of the body.

Continuing down the leg, the channel has many points alongside the fibula. Before it crosses over the ankle just above its lateral prominence, it passes down into the foot. Here we find Gall Bladder 41, Foot Overlooking Tears. This point is related to Gall Bladder 15, Head Overlooking Tears, and like that point can assist in promoting or slowing down tears. It is also the opening point for the *dai mai* or belt vessel named the Vessel of Latency. Latency refers to all those potentials that reside within us, some we have stuffed deep inside us to hold on to dearly. It is fitting that this point of the Gall Bladder channel can be used to help release pent-up energies and get them flowing again.

An additional aspect of the Gall Bladder worth noting at this point and in direct relationship to its position in the sides of the legs is the role of lateral stabilization. When going this way and that, we must lean right and left with the winds as they blow, like the ship at sea.

In order to keep a true course and not capsize or waver along the way, our lateral stabilizers must be strong and vital. This description is an apt metaphor for the work of the Gall Bladder in the body, heart-mind, and spirit.

From 41, Foot Overlooking Tears, the channel travels on between the bones of the fourth and fifth toe to find its termination at the base of the nail of the fourth toe. Resting here after its long traverse of the body with its wild tracing from front to back to front to back to front to back, its job of distributing energies throughout the body is finally accomplished.

Liver Meridian

Foot Jue Yin

Here we find the expression of Jue Yin in the lower body. Between the Kidney and the Spleen we find the Liver. The Kidney is the most deep in the Shao Yin layer, the Spleen is the most superficial as Tai Yin and the

Liver is in the middle as Jue Yin. Understanding the relative relation to the outside world of each of these organs, this makes a degree of sense. The spleen/pancreas is directly related to interfacing with food as it first comes into the body via saliva and enzymatic secretions in the digestive track.

The liver is deeper still with its involvement in the inner workings of blood sugar, creating cellular food from absorbed nutrients, dealing with detoxification and all the many chemical equations the liver deals with in the physiology of the body. The kidney is deeper still, working directly with the blood and vascular system.

Wood Element

The middle yin function is linked to the Wood element's organization distribution, reliability, and integrity. It is said that the Liver is in charge of the smooth flow of qi throughout the human body. We could see this as analogous to the gentle breezes of the atmosphere caused by high and low pressure systems working in an integrated fashion all around the globe. Anything jagged or stormy brings a challenge to the smooth conduct of affairs, but fair weather and a good breeze mean for smooth and steady sailing on the seas of life.

1 to 3 am

Here in the very darkest hours of the night, we find the Liver channel most alive and vital. It is in these overnight hours when much is digested and completed as we dream. It is said in the classics that the eyes are the sprout of the Liver and that vision is the sense most closely related to Liver function. And it is not merely physical visual acuity that is at stake here but rather the whole of the visionary process.

The hours of 1 to 3 am is the dream time, the time for a deeper vision of our life and purpose. For many a college student this is the term paper hour. The parties have finally ended; only the die-hards are still at it. The procrastinators facing imminent deadlines finally have to crank out those last ten pages of content and crunch that last bit of data to present a complete project or paper. The quiet of this time serves to support this most important task.

Key Functions
Planning center, central storehouse

Affirmation
I envision my life with clarity and purpose.

The Liver channel of Foot Jue Yin begins in the big toe and ends in the torso just below the breast. It has been characterized in the classics as the general in charge of the troops, responsible for their conduct. Its primary range of functions is in planning and storage, and it is responsible for myriad functions in body, heartmind, and spirit. As such we find that it is responsible for the smooth and integrated interrelationship of all the energies of our lives. More details of its physical, mental, emotional, and spiritual range of functions are found in the descriptions below.

Key Characteristics of the Functional Range of the Liver Channel
Physical
At the physical level the liver performs the functions of storing and releasing blood sugars, transmuting nutrient intake into cellular level foods needed by all the systems of the body. Further, the liver creates bile for the breaking down of fats into fuel. It detoxifies the blood and body, taking any toxins that invade the body and converting them to useful material or working to eliminate them from the body. And it does all this in a timely manner.

Due to its important task of fueling the body, liver function is directly related to our stamina and energy supply. It performs the role of storing blood sugars, converting them into cell food, and dispersing that fuel to the body on an as needed basis. Because of the cyclic nature of life and demands, the liver works in a cyclic manner in its management of the body's energy storehouse.

The liver has long been known as the organ in charge of detoxification. The liver clears toxic matter from the body; an overabundance of intoxicants can damage the liver. The classic Chinese texts correlate the Liver network to the eyes, and indeed we find that various liver conditions such as jaundice present symptoms in the eyes. Tears produced when crying have been found to clear the body of toxins, making crying a vital way for the Liver to detoxify the body.

The Liver is directly involved with masculine potency, as impotence is often a result of fatigue and stress on the Liver. Restoring Liver function plays a vital role in maintaining virility for men.

PSYCHOLOGICAL, EMOTIONAL

Moving beyond the physical level of functioning into the levels of the psychological and emotional realms, we see Liver functioning as the visionary planner. As we mentioned above, the eyes are said to be the sprout of the Liver, but deeper than any physical aspect of vision, the eyes are a metaphor for the vision we hold for our lives and what our lives are about. The Liver is critical in this function, and its health is of utmost importance in supporting the clarity of our vision. A good cry is said to be cleansing to the Liver, and it often happens in relation to those things for which we care most deeply.

Crying is indeed a powerful aid in detoxification, and after cleansing our vision through our tears we can see the path that lies ahead clearly.

With all its many responsibilities to keep the body running, the Liver channel is responsible for the smooth flow of energy throughout the body, a process that manifests in smooth body movements, easy emotions, and a steady, calm attitude when faced with changes or challenges.

Whenever we experience spasticity or sharp and dramatic emotions, it is the Liver calling out for help.

The Liver is often described as the chief executive officer, called upon to always have the answer and know what's best.

Sometimes its direction can feel controlling, and indeed its job is to keep control though the occasional power play may be involved to keep the upper hand in any situation.

This type of control can often be accompanied by deep ingrained habits, in musculature and in the architecture of mental attitudes. The Liver can manifest as the trustworthy person in control or the control freak subject to falling into addictive tendencies.

Any habit of body or mind that becomes an obsession can be related to Liver energy. And with it can come powerful bursts of emotion, anger, shouting, and screaming that can all be gone with the next breath.

SPIRITUAL

The highest application of a capable Liver is a steady hand on the tiller; wise, knowing, and clear-sighted. The Liver concerns itself spiritually with matters of higher life purpose and spiritual vision.

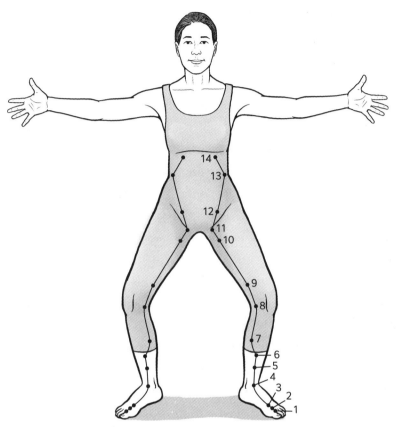

Figure 14: Liver Meridian—Foot Jue Yin.

1. Great Pile
2. Between Columns
3. Great Rushing
4. Middle Seal
5. Shell Groove
6. Middle Capital
7. Knee Pass

8. Spring at the Bend
9. Yin Envelope
10. Leg Five Miles
11. Yin Screen
12. Rapid Pulse
13. Camphorwood Gate
14. Gate of the Cycle

The Liver Channel Trajectory

As Gall Bladder completes its journey, it passes the baton to its yin partner, the Liver. From the fourth toe, the energy of the one meridian crosses over to the top of the big toe where the Liver energy first manifests on the surface of the body. The big toe is the first to test the water, an action illustrative of the Liver's job in assessing the feasibility of any plan. Along with the second toe, the big toe is also the first part of the body to move ahead and push off into the unknown. As we've explored already, the healthier the Liver, the more confident the stride.

From the great toe, the Liver pathway continues up through the valley between the first and second toe where we find Liver 3, Great Rushing. The name elicits a connection to the Liver's function. The big toe must work very hard to maintain our stability and keep us moving forward. As we rush or surge forward into the world, the big toe leads the way and the Liver is the mastermind behind it all.

After Liver 3 the channel moves up the foot and passes through the ankle's anterior medial aspect. It travels back to connect with its yin leg meridian partners at Spleen 6, Three Yin Meeting. It then returns to the front, rising along the medial edge of the shin bone until about halfway between the ankle and the knee. Here it travels toward the back of the leg, crossing over the Spleen meridian, finding its line of travel parallel to and between the Spleen and the Kidney meridians. In this most medial position of the leg it crosses the inner knee where we find Liver 8, Spring at the Bend. This name has a beautiful double meaning as both a spring like flowing water and flexibility at the knee joint. Like a tennis player moving back and forth across the court to keep the volley alive, the necessity for springy knees is essential. The Wood element also governs all sinew action, important in joint mobilization in general and in the knee in particular.

The Liver channel then rises up the inner thigh along the adductor muscles and into the groin. Here it traverses the powerful muscles guarding and managing the reproductive zone in all its functions, a quality that speaks to the Liver's role in fertility. We store the energy necessary to propagate the species and simultaneously maintain the capacity to plan adequately for new members of the human race to be brought into the world.

Passing through the inguinal canal, the channel veers out to the sides where it touches the tip of the twelfth rib at Liver 13, Camphorwood Gate. This point is the alarm point for the Spleen/Pancreas, and its position on the Liver meridian speaks of supporting the right relationship between Wood and Earth.

The ancient proverb reads: "Where the Wood meets the Earth, there rises a thousand pieces of valuable timber." Camphorwood in particular is a very precious wood that has a value of mythical proportions.

Finally, Liver turns toward the front once more where it finds its ending point in the sixth intercostal space at Liver 14, Gate of the Cycle. This point is directly in line with and just two ribs below the nipple. Its name speaks to the completion of the daily cycle and also speaks to anything in our lives where we need to manifest a feeling of completion. In fact, an alternate name for the point is Completion Gate.

To be able to say that we have realized our vision and achieved our goals having completed each step is a vital aspect to which Liver 14 relates. From here the energy rises to meet the Lung channel and the cycle continues for as long as there is life flowing in the body.

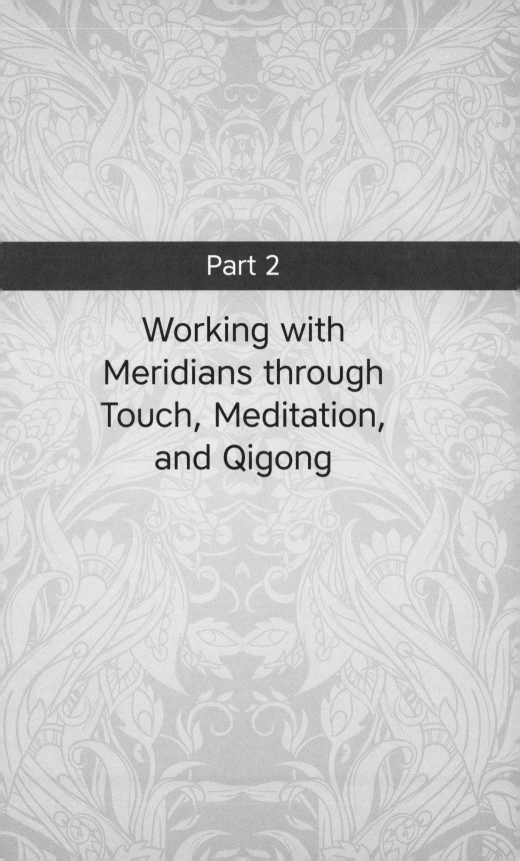

Part 2

Working with Meridians through Touch, Meditation, and Qigong

With a working knowledge of the meridian functions, locations, and important points along each channel, you are now equipped with a treasure trove of information on how your body works and how it is organized. All the working parts of your body and their many and various ways of interacting with one another can keep you balanced, healthy, and vivacious for years to come. In this section we will begin the work of crafting this knowedge into a set of practical working exercises to help you on your way to greater balance, harmony, and ease.

Generally, all these parts of your being are extremely intelligent and do their job unerringly for years on end. But there are times when we all fall down, systems seem to fail, something goes wrong, and we find ourselves off track. Balance is elusive and vitality is scarce. That's when we need some skillful intervention to support the body and its many functions. Particularly important is to be able to locate where the distress is most prominent and help to restore balance once more.

The knowledge of meridian functions, locations, and active points is valuable, but what is more important is to have ways of entering with consciousness to assess and treat your body's energetic system when it is in need. With thirty years of working with the body using these tools and thousands of years of healing tradition behind me, I will guide you through powerful tools you can use to help yourself into better balance.

I'm going to explore with you a range of approaches, from meditation and movement to healing touch. These are time-honored tools that have effectively helped thousands, and I use them myself on a daily basis with great results that keep me fit and functional. There's no magic bullet here, mind you, but these approaches are remarkably effective and can help you resolve many difficult situations when practiced with diligence.

As you work with these tools, I remind you that these methods are not a substitute for professional medical care. They are not meant to diagnose or treat serious conditions, and if you find that your body simply is not responding with noticeable improvement, you are encouraged to consult your physician.

In addition, I have several training programs across the United States. I have personally trained hundreds of students to a professional level and their support may be vital to you. Also, as director of education for the American Organization for Bodywork Therapies of Asia, I am in close contact with dozens of highly trained professionals in Asian Bodywork Therapy all over the world. You'll find my contact information in the back of this book, and I'll be happy to hear from you and support you in any way I can. You may wish to pursue training yourself and take the work within these pages deeper with expert in-person guidance.

For now, practice what is taught here and begin to learn for yourself the value and applications of *Pathways of Qi*'s knowledge and technique. When you are ready to go deeper and join a live training, you will know. Meanwhile, all the techniques recommended in this book are safe and effective for home use. As with any such approach, remember that words and pictures in a book can set you on the right path and begin the process, but ultimately an in-person training session will be the most effective way to embody the practice.

Remember, you are your own authority. You have lived in your body your entire life, an experience neither I nor any other teacher have. You will be the one who ultimately decides if any given technique or approach works for you and at what level of depth or intensity. If anything is beyond your capacity, don't do it! If you don't feel you are being pushed hard enough, increase the intensity slowly and carefully.

What follows are time-honored techniques that may at first seem simplistic or even boring. You will not find power gymnastics nor power yoga in these pages. The art of working with qi is an art of consciousness more than physical exercise. In fact, benefits are often derived more from doing less and paying attention more. In the end, these are more arts of being than arts of doing: the less you do, the more you actually achieve.

An important principle of practice is known as the 70/30 rule. Following this principle in your practice, you only ever use 70 percent of your energy in any given task and at the same time can keep 30 percent in reserve. The wisdom suggests that by keeping 30 percent in resereve, you will always have something left to give in the case of an emergency. It may seem to run counter to the usual Western admonition to give 110 percent; in many ways it does. But don't in any way think it is inferior. With cultivation, your 70 percent may soon exceed another person's 110 percent and you'll still have 30 percent in reserve, just in case.

Take this admonition to heart and see if it can help you to hone your practice of awakening the flow of qi through your own meridian pathways. What this ultimatley can create for you is a state of ease and flow. Making certain to eliminate force, and connect with a flow greater than your own skill could ever manufacture on its own is the key.

If you should have any questions along the way, as revelations arise from your practice of the application of these methods, please check the resource section in the back of this book for details on how to contact me or other qualified trainers in the field. I'll be happy to help you find the answers you are seeking and realize the ways these methods can support you on your way.

Chapter 8

Assessing and Working with Meridians

Learning to work with meridians begins with studying the centered, balanced, and healthy expression of each channel. From there it progresses to learning to discern the continuum of presentations that can express themselves when an imbalance is settling into place. For instance, the Lung channel governs our experience of gain and loss and the many complex expressions of grief. If the Lung is balanced, we may find that we can take things in stride and roll with life's gains and losses with authenticity, proper concern, and alacrity. But if the Lung is compromised in any way we can blow things off, deny the pain, and move on without having ever really dealt with it, or on the opposite end of the spectrum could get lost in our pool of grief and find that it renders us dysfunctional for an extended period. All the channels can demonstrate these wide swings, and learning to assess our energy at any given point in our lives is key to maintaining or restoring healthy functionality. In this chapter we'll investigate the basic tools for assessing a systemic state of balance.

Harmonizing Qi Energy

To harmonize life energy in the whole being, it is vital to have an appreciation for patterns of harmony and disharmony. The Three Treasures as the body's fundamental substances can be perceived qualitatively and quantitatively. When in balance they together express harmony, whereas a predominance of one over the others or various deficiencies can lead to disharmony. A primary tool for identifying such patterns is the ability to read signs and feel for the presence of excess or deficiency in the body's qi. The late Master Masunaga, a twentieth-century Japanese shiatsu therapist who became famous for his method, Zen Shiatsu, had an elegant way of describing excess and deficiency. In the touch therapy world of Asian bodywork therapy, it became known as the kyo jitsu theory.

For fifteen years, I trained and taught at the Ohashi Institute where the Masunaga kyo jitsu theory was at the core of our healing touch training. I have taught this model to thousands and use it effectively and regularly in my own clinical practice. When working with the pathways of qi, it is a powerful ally in working to harmonize qi in the body, heartmind, and spirit. Presented here is the foundation to understanding kyo jitsu so this profound approach can deepen your own practice and experience.

Kyo and *jitsu* describe two states of energy expression found in an overall pattern of energy distortion. Distorted or imbalanced energy states are called *jyaki*, literally "distorted ki." (*Ki* is the Japanese pronunciation of the Chinese *qi*.) Within the distortion are two distinct aspects, the deficiency and the excess. *Kyo* is the term describing the deficient condition; *jitsu* describes any excess.

In true yin/yang fashion, kyo and jitsu do not exist one without the other and always manifest in relationship to one another. In Western terms we call this a compensatory system. When one aspect of any system goes into deficiency, another will go into overdrive in order to compensate.

To bring this squarely into our discussion, kyo and jitsu describe qi as it manifests in the meridian pathways. As one example of a disharmonious pattern, think of someone who has a massive appetite but not much emotional sensitivity. Such a person would be manifesting what we would call a Stomach jitsu with a Heart kyo. You can see how this could lead to misfortune and suffering if it were to go on for too long. And while the appetite for food and stimulation might be served, the deeper need for tender loving care could be long unmet and lead to serious problems.

According to Masuanaga's clinical observations kyo is the cause and jitsu the result. Another way of saying that would be kyo as the need and jitsu as the action to fill the need. Kyo is often difficult to see but jitsu shows up because it is action oriented. You may not be able to see that a person is hungry, but the way in which they go about looking for food or preparing and eating the food will be the action that tips you off to the underlying hunger as the motivating factor. To continue with this example, you could also see that a massive appetite (Stomach jitsu) is a compensation for the true need—love and connection (Heart kyo).

It is important to note that identifying kyo and jitsu is not about finding out what is wrong with you; rather it is seeking to discover what is right with you. It is natural to have needs and take action to fulfill them; this is true on the level of the entire organism as a whole as well as for each individual organ system in its own domain. For instance the Stomach has a need to feed the body and will compel the body into action to fulfill that need. Thank God! If you are hungry, you need to eat. The hope is that you will have access to good, nutritious food to truly fulfill your body's need for fuel. So too does the Heart have a need for order, safety, intimacy, and love. When those things are lacking, promptings toward actions that could lead to fulfillment will happen.

A properly identified need leads to an appropriate action to find fulfillment when things proceed in a balanced manner. Yet as we know from life, it is often easier said than done. All too often we have misidentified our needs and taken actions that could likely be wildly off the mark. Such actions fail to fill the true need and also create a whole set of conditions that create new needs. Take for instance our example of Stomach jitsu and Heart kyo. If the true need is for love, affection, and a sense of belonging and the only thing you have at hand is a box of cookies, your need for love will likely be mitigated for the time being but the true need will still exist. Here we find ourselves heading down the path to jyaki—distorted, imbalanced qi. Too many nights assuaging your need for love with the cookie jar will lead to a serious state of imbalance.

To properly restore balance, we have several possible approaches. The first and foremost understanding is that if we can properly identify the need and properly meet it with right action, the need will be fulfilled and balance restored. Doing so helps us be in good balance the next time a need arises and a new right action is undertaken to fulfill it. When kyo is fulfilled or satisfied, we call this tonification. Tonification is considered the ultimate cure for imbalance, because once a true deficiency has been satisfied, all the mistaken jitsu actions that were attempting to fulfill that need cease.

What I've just described of course is a perfect world. More realistically, our jitsu actions continue sometimes out of force of habit and continually conspire to throw the system out of balance and create new needs for re-correction. In such a case it can become necessary to rein in misguided jitsu actions through a method known as sedation. Sedation is generally considered a more aggressive intervention and is therefore somewhat dangerous, but generally it leads to a quick cessation of the immediate offending influence.

Let's explore an example of this so you can have a more complete picture. Consider an "empty marriage," where a husband has an insatiable sexual appetite and the wife is estranged. The husband engages in extra-marital affairs while away on business trips. Though estranged, the wife is understandably and justifiably hurt by her husband's breaking of their vows when she finds out about the affairs. Imagine that the wife responds by having a romantic affair of her own with a colleague in her professional life. Sadly, in her attempt to get back at her errant husband, she nearly destroys her own career. Clearly the need to connect and achieve true satisfying intimacy within their marital commitment is shattered.

Now here is where sophisticated intervention on the part of someone skilled in reading the excess and deficiency patterns truly helps. As long as the damage isn't beyond repair and there is a sincere commitment on the part of the husband and wife to mend their marriage, skillful intervention to identify the true need and apply a compassionate approach with commitments on both sides through a series of trust building assignments could well help this couple overcome over their struggles and build a deeply satisfying relationship.

In this case a combination of sedation and tonification is necessary. Both husband and wife need to constrain their jitsu actions. They need to begin to talk honestly and rebuild trust in one another; tonifying their true needs, in short. If they succeed in rebuilding the lost relationship, they ultimately satisfy their true deep need for intimacy and contact.

Perhaps this can best be summarized in Leon Hammer's words: "We all need contact. Enough contact to remain intact. In the absence of positive contact, negative contact will do. And in the worst case scenario, negative contact becomes a way of life."[2] Our job then in healing this pattern is to conspire to create and maintain positive contact in all our relationships with humans and nature. This can be arduous work but in the end it is the only work worth doing.

---

2   Leon Hammer, *Dragon Rises, Red Bird Flies* (Seattle: Eastland Press, 2005), 47.

Learning to use the kyo jistu model with its proper applications of tonification and sedation can bring about deeply positive and lasting change in our lives. The garden of life can flourish and become abundantly productive. Properly identify your needs and the needs of each organ system and you will make choices for action in the world that fulfill your highest good and the highest good for everyone with whom you are in contact.

Rather than simply perpetuating your old ways of doing things out of habit and misguided thinking, cultivate compassion and see all your actions as a cry for help, a call to note your deeper needs, and a chance to realize true fulfillment one need at a time. This is not to say that all your needs will ever be met or completely satisfied; on the contrary, need is ever present. One could even say that need is everything. Indeed it is the driving force that makes life itself unfold. Our goal is not to eradicate need but to embrace it. When we can embrace our needs, we can take appropriate action to fulfill them, and in their fulfillment find ourselves stronger and more confident to meet all our needs as they arise.

When applying the kyo jitsu model to the meridian system, through inquiry and touch, you can read the quality of the qi energy within each meridian channel. Then you can treat the kyo and jitsu qualities at the energetic level, tonifying the deficiency and sedating the excess to restore balance within the system. The art of this method is based on the realization that imbalance shows up early in the body on subtle levels; once you've learned to read those subtle energetic signs, you can apply proper corrections at an early stage in the development of any pattern of imbalance, thus preventing it from manifesting in a more serious fashion.

There are many methods employed in the work of establishing and maintaining equilibrium within the meridian system. Exercise, meditation, and proper diet are the first order of business in self-care. Following that, the external supports of counseling and coaching through skilled therapeutic touch, exercise physiology, and psychological and spiritual counseling. If further need exists, we have the entire tool kit of the modern healing arts practitioner ranging from the needles, herbs, and supplements of the acupuncture doctor to the pharmaceutical and surgical interventions of the Western medical professional. In the latter, we face the problem that most Western-trained physicians are either unaware of, unconvinced of the presence and validity of the meridian system. With training and understanding, these physicians can learn to be sensitive to the signs and clues of the body's energy system and thus improve the quality of their care with a whole new set of tools for assessment and treatment.

On the topic of interventions, we must recognize that this too is an action to meet a need. The proper identification of the need and the appropriate application of effort to meet it still remain at the core of the journey. Doctors can be misguided in their interventions just as an individual might be in attempts at self-correction. Though through a well-informed and educated position we can all hone our interventions to a higher level. We must proceed with utmost care and compassion, equipping ourselves with the best of knowledge and understanding, and only then can we proceed down the road to establishing, supporting, and maintaining harmony and balance in our lives and the lives of those we serve.

Looking at Assessment and Treatment Strategies

If you have a desire to work with your meridian energy or even become a therapist and use your knowledge of meridians to help others, you must develop skillful ways of assessment and treatment. In this work I will explore touch therapy (this chapter), exercise (chapter 10), and meditation (chapter 9) as the primary method of treatment, but there are a wide range of treatment strategies and likely some combination of approaches will be important for healing in most cases. The ancient Chinese texts mention regions of the kingdom where methods of treatment arose. In the east they became wise in the use of food; in the south, herbal remedies were developed; in the west, exercise was central to maintaining good health; in the north they discovered acupuncture; and in the center of the land, touch therapy was developed. Each and every one of these approaches is efficacious and should have a place in your tool kit.

As we explore assessment and treatment strategies it is of utmost importance to remember that assessment is treatment and treatment is assessment. While you are in the process of observing and assessing a situation's energetic balance, you are also affecting that situation. While you are treating and intentionally affecting the energetic system, you must assess as you go along to read the quality of your intervention, and track progress of changes toward balance and harmony. I will explore assessment in this light, and then enter into a discussion of treatment strategies based on ongoing awareness of assessment principles.

In assessment methods our first exploration must be philosophical, to understand the agreements one must hold in the work of helping yourself and another. What's essential here is to see that we progress in a practical way, not simply dogmatically or because the book said so. Our efforts must, as Sun Bear was known to say, "grow corn." This is not some philosophy for erudite scholars in some out-of-this-world location—it is practical, day-to-day material that improves our lives.

The Four Methods of Assessment

To begin, let's explore what are known as the four methods of assessment: observation, inquiry, listening, and touching. Simple in their practical nature, these methods ask us to improve our ability to be aware and perceive in some detail whatever we are presented. A certain ability to read signs and symptoms is required and from those observations to extrapolate suppositions as to what the signs and symptoms portend.

Observation is the first method. In observation it is essential that we come from a neutral place. In other words, we must not actively scan in such a way as to be overly specific in our efforts. Rather it is suggested that you even allow your gaze to become a bit fuzzy, step back, and take in the general picture first. When you are looking at yourself, this can be rather tricky. Honest self-evaluation can be elusive, and the lack of an objective viewpoint not only makes your vision a bit fuzzy, but downright obscured. In this case you may want to enlist the help of trusted friends and confidants for some honest reflection. When doing this work it is of utmost importance to not fall into shame and blame, or making anything out to be wrong, but rather always to look with an eye to supporting and giving service in the name of growth and greater awareness. When observing another person you also don't want to go about making the person uncomfortable, or self-conscious to the idea that they are being scrutinized. Instead, look by not looking, observe without making a point of observing. Simply open your awareness to what is being revealed to you.

By allowing yourself to become fully present and receptive to whatever shows up, you remove any pre-supposed ideas that could actually cloud your ability to see what is really going on. You also place whomever you're observing at ease, so that they will be more likely to show up truthfully and honestly. Remember, in the end it is not what is wrong with you, but what is right with you, that we are seeking. And an honest open attentiveness to whatever shows up is the correct and most productive attitude to cultivate.

Inquiry is a vast and far-reaching art. Your ability to ask a question is key in revealing the most important aspect of any situation. To ask in the proper frame of mind is to ask with complete curiosity about the answer. Presumptions limit the quality of an inquiry tremendously. Make your questions honest and clear, and let them arise from your clear desire to get to know the situation without judgment. There is a level of questioning that can be free of judgment and also lead you down a specific path, following up on hunches you may have received from your observations or the answers to previous questions.

In her seminal work, *All Sickness is Homesickness* (1994), author Dianne Connely suggests learning to ask the "home run question," the question that brings us all home.[3] If we are sick, it is a sign of an estrangement from our true nature. What has led us astray may be that which ultimately will point the way home. We go off in pursuit of something each time we take a step. Do you know where you are going and what you are looking for?

Take a step back and ask yourself a compassionate question: Can you see in the undertaking of all of your actions in the world (jitsu) your sincere intent to meet your needs (kyo)? Even though your action may not be skillful or miss the mark, can you see that your choices can reveal more and more information to you about your deeper needs you are working to fulfill? When helping a friend or a client, can you take a path of inquiry that tracks their experiences and choices to the source of their motivation? Perhaps an underlying belief is running the show, but that belief is false or at least no longer valid. If you see someone behaving badly to get attention, can you get past the bad behavior and help reveal the true need for attention underneath that behavior? If you can do that, it's possible to solve the problem of the bad behavior by simply asking the right question. And asking the right question can lead you to true answers that will bring forth great healing.

Listening is the third method, related to inquiry. Listening is the art of hearing not just the words that are spoken but also the tone of voice and whatever else is not stated explicitly. Some call it reading between the lines, but it is in no way meant to present yourself as superior or knowing better; simply, you open yourself up to messages that come in the silence between the words. A good assessment is based on careful listening. It's often when someone realizes they are actually being listened to with care

---

3   Dianne Connelley, *All Sickness Is Home Sickness* (Columbia, MD: Wisdom Well Press, 1993), 71.

and interest that they will in turn open themselves up to share more honestly and completely than ever in their lives. Become a good listener and you will become excellent at assessment. Don't listen for what you want to hear, listen to what is being said and how.

Touch is the final confirmation of what you have been observing, inquiring after, and listening for. Touching is an expression of contact that yields in-depth and immediate information. More information actually comes in than you might ever actually be able to be conscious of. In touch, it's as if all the other methods are rolled into one. You observe, ask, and listen at each point of contact. Ask: "What does the body tissue have to say to me? How does it respond to my touch? Does it yearn for deeper pressure, or lighter pressure, or longer or shorter contact?" Ask these questions aloud as you touch; listen for the tissue to respond. Is it uptight or relaxed? Is the person liking what you are doing or recoiling or flinching? Does it feel like you are invited to stay longer, or is it hoped you'll go away soon? Is it weak or strong? Here we begin to feel the actual qualities of kyo and jitsu—the deplete and the replete, the empty, needy cold, or the full saturated, hot. Open your perception with touch and you will find a nearly instinctive ability to read the response of the person to your contact. Perception will guide you to offering the best service possible, tailored to meet the needs of the person just as you find them.

As you grow with these four methods and you marry them to a deepening understanding of the qi energy matrix of the body, heartmind, and spirit, your observations, inquiry, listening, and touching will come alive with information and fascination. You will have entered the realm of true human contact at the very deepest level and open the doorway to deep and lasting healing. These four methods will lead you to the channels most crying out for help and guide your treatment strategy to meet the emergent needs of the person with whom you are in contact.

When we use touch to assess the quality of qi in any given point or pathway, there are certain cues to identifying kyo/deficient and jitsu/excess conditions. Once you have gained proficiency at identifying these, you will have a good idea of whether to proceed with tonification or sedation methods. Remember, tonification is used to support and reenergize a deficiency, while sedation or dispersal is used to reduce an excess condition. If the basic understanding of kyo and jitsu is unclear, go back and review the foundation material in the earlier section, "Harmonizing Qi Energy." The rest of this discussion builds upon the understanding established there.

First we think of kyo as the need and jitsu as the action to fill the need. We also see kyo as emptiness and jitsu as fullness. Since the two words are used to describe the quality of qi energy in a given meridian channel, it would stand to reason that the actual tissue along the pathway of the meridian will feel one way when it is kyo and another way when it is jitsu. The question then becomes, what does needy, empty feel like, and how does that compare to active, fullness? One of the key factors that shows up at the tissue layer is what we call resiliency. Does the tissue bounce back when you press it, or is it non-responsive, either flaccid or taut?

Healthy tissue is resilient, having a natural give and take, and it is appropriately responsive to the quality of touch given. Kyo tissue will tend to be flat in response and not fight back at all. In fact, it tends to give way, like you're falling in to a deep chasm. Jitsu tissue on the other hand will be taut like piano wire or a flat board; it will seem to fight and not let you in at all.

There are many ways to describe the feel of kyo and jitsu. One of the more sensitive guiding questions in touch therapy is "Does it call you in or push you away?" The answer to this question sometimes has little to do with actual tissue resiliency and much to do with a sense of inner knowing that you develop over time. It is at least in part innate.

When someone is open to your touch, it is made clear to you in many ways; when a person is not open to it, there is just as clear an indication that this is the case. As you develop your sensitivity, you will learn to validate your felt sense of responsiveness at this level. It is fascinating to explore and respond to this information.

Interpreting the Body's Messages

What's important to understand here is that the human body energetically is both a transmitter and receiver. As a transmitter it is constantly putting out signals to the world that broadcast the content of its programming. As a receiver it is sensitive to picking up the signals from other beings and listening to what they are putting out over the airwaves. When you learn to tune into the frequency of another human being or to the different aspects of your own being, you are cultivating your assessment abilities. You can learn to know when some part is crying out for help or when it is manifesting dissonance. At the same time, you can learn to read when it is in a state of harmony and ease. As you attune your sensitivity, you will begin to identify the clues which point toward kyo conditions which are asking for tonification, as compared to jitsu conditions which call for restraint or dispersal.

Pain as Signal

Everyone has a certain relationship with pain. We all feel it from time to time, sometimes intensely, sometimes mildly. One Chinese system differentiates between fifty kinds of pain, suggesting that it is in the proper identification of the pain signal that one can hit upon the correct treatment strategy. One kind of pain calls for intensification, taking the pain sensation even more deeply in order to release it. Another calls for backing off and breathing gently and deeply. Some pain would best be treated with encouraging you to scream and cry and pound your fists into a pillow. Still others are greeted with silence and introspection.

This is a deep art that's highly individualized, so it is important not to overgeneralize or try on a one-size-fits-all model. For many of us, our own intuitive understanding about how to work with our pain is generally the correct one. Sometimes the most effective approach may prove counterintuitive, in which case there is nothing that can replace the assistance of a skilled practitioner. Until you can find such skilled support the general rule of thumb is to try an approach, see how it works, and keep going if it yields beneficial results. If it seems to lead nowhere or makes things significantly worse, stop and try something else.

To fully teach the intricacies of intuitive pain treatment is simply beyond the scope of this book; only individualized in-person treatment will do. But it is important here to understand that pain and all bodily sensations come in many forms and levels—one would do well not to think in overly simplistic terms about pain signals we receive. To simply reach for the aspirin or Tylenol or some stronger medication when feeling an uncomfortable sensation is a short-sighted strategy. Even putting pain on a scale of one to ten is only just a start. Rather, begin to understand that pain is a signal, the body is crying out for attention. We must not seek to mask it or make it wrong, but rather open up to it, listen to it, and see if we can figure out what it is trying to tell us. To that end, let's explore a few different variations and strategies for using pain signals as an interpretive tool.

Redefining Pain as Specific Sensations

First I wish to engage the idea of redefining and even eliminating the use of the word *pain*. As a word, pain is not very descriptive. Really, it's a negative judgment about a sensation and not the feeling itself. Pain is such a general idea that its meaning may be diluted to the point of uselessness. In general, we could say that pain is all those feelings that we don't particularly like. And pain exists in contrast to pleasure, all those sensations that we do like. As such, it is a useful term only for determining the rough category of our reaction to what we are feeling.

One other possibility for seeing the place of pain is that it can generally be used as an indication that something is out of balance in the system, kind of like a warning light in an automobile. But we need to be careful here; we often fall into the trap that if we feel pain there must be something wrong with us. Remember the overriding philosophy of our inquiry must be the question "What is right with me?" not "What is wrong with me?" Whether painful or pleasurable, sensations coming from our body all carry a message to us about the nature of our experience in the body at this time. The work is to open up to the sensation so we can listen to the message.

To do so, we must reorient ourselves to get past the idea that something is painful and instead enter the realm of describing the exact nature of the sensation we are interpreting as pain. In order to understand the feeling that we are having, we must get beyond the judgmental mind that says "I feel good" or "I feel bad" and describe what exactly it is that we are feeling. We will probably find that there are not only fifty kinds of pain (or pleasure, for that matter), but an infinite variety of sensations all of differing quality.

Here is a list of sensations and feelings that could serve as a starting place for this inquiry. The idea here is that if I am describing my sensations, anyone listening can have a direct appreciation with little interpretation about what it is I'm feeling.

Warm, cold, hot, tingling, pins and needles, achy, sore, dull, sharp, stuck, soft, weak, hard, tight, strong, searing, shooting, throbbing, undulating, buzzing, heavy, light, weird, normal, itchy, hungry, full, numb, empty, dark, dry, wet, juicy, rigid, flaccid, limp, sleepy, twitchy, quiet, loud, fixed, moving, alive, dead, open, closed, big, vast, small, tiny.

This list is in no way exhaustive, but it should give you an idea of some useful terminology to begin to enter into a description of the actual sensations you are feeling in your body. The list also exposes the indicators or the kyo and jitsu aspect of our dialogue with our bodily sensations, giving us an idea of the vocabulary necessary for interpreting the message of our bodily signals. Our dialogue is guided by a recognition of opposites. Hot or cold? Tight or loose? Weird or normal? Awake or sleepy? Moving or stuck? These oppositions are a basic indicator of yang and yin, jitsu and kyo, bringing us back to the understanding of where we are in the ongoing natural cycle of change from yin to yang and yang to yin.

As you begin to practice this method of perceiving the sensations in your body, you will find that they change and shift sometimes subtly, sometimes dramatically. Take your time, slow down, and be receptive. Reduce your reactivity and the fear that something is wrong—just listen. In listening, you may receive a message and discover what your body wisdom is telling you. In working with others, you can slow them down and guide them to the practice of describing their sensations. You'll gain valuable insight into the exact nature of just what they are going through, and you can respond appropriately.

A simple inquiry into the quality of so-called pain or the sensation of discomfort and its response to touch is valuable here. Some "pains" will be relieved when touched, others will intensify upon contact. If the sensation is saying, "Ooh, yes, please rub there, please go deeper," this is generally considered an indication of a kyo condition. It is calling you in. If the response is "Ouch! Stop it! That hurts!" this is an indication of a jitsu condition. It is pushing you away. Together we call them the "hurt so good, hurt so bad" clues to kyo and jitsu.

So in these ways, we can begin to shape our understanding of pain or discomfort, and beyond that all our sensations as indicators of kyo and jitsu conditions of the energy field. Ultimately, the determination of kyo or jitsu is a process of developing your felt sense and trusting your inner knowingness. There is nothing you can do to force the feelings; you simply need to open up, get out of your head, and become openly attentive to whatever arises.

From Assessment to Treatment

From assessment to treatment we engage in an interesting journey. Remember that ultimately, in these arts, assessment is treatment, treatment is assessment. You cannot look, ask, listen, and touch without also effecting some change in the body, heartmind, and spirit. Likewise, as you are effecting change, you must be "assessing" the nature of that change as you go along. This all sounds pretty heady, but ultimately it is not an intellectual exercise. Remember, there is no separation between feelings and the intellect. Just be aware that there really is no objective reality. We are all engaged in the deep interactive process of movement and change called living. Jump in with both feet and hands, and have some fun.

Once we have all these clues into the nature of kyo and jitsu as well as a knowledge of the meridian locations, points, and functions, we can begin the process of pattern distinction or recognition. The inquiry becomes directed toward the questions: "Where in the body, heartmind. and spirit are the kyo and jistu conditions most clear?" "Which meridian function is most calling out for help?" In establishing a baseline of understanding about where the system is in its cycle of changes you can make a call as to what would be the most effective intervention to assist the optimal functioning. To this end develop your understanding of functions and characteristics of the channels as a guide to assisting in the maintenance of balance in the system.

The methods of treatment grow out of the methods of assessment. Once you have established your recognition of the kyo and jitsu aspects, you respond to these with tonification and sedation. Tonification is the process of building the kyo, nurturing and meeting the true need. Sedation is the process of dispersing, dissipating, or restraining an excess condition. In using touch therapy, tonification is generally a slow, gentle, deeply nurturing contact, whereas sedation is a stronger, quicker more agitating contact.

For a deeper exploration of therapeutic touch approaches, there are many training manuals that guide you through the shiatsu and other compatible touch therapies like massage or acupressure that may use the meridian channels to increase the treatment's effectiveness. I personally conduct and ultimately recommend live training in any touch therapy, as it is the only way to receive adequate training in any craft. In the meantime, get started with the exercises taught here, and see to what end you can make positive change as you follow these instructions. There are many ways in which you can practice tonification and sedation on your own through brushing and tapping, meditation, and qigong exercises. And you may also find skilled nutritionists and herbalists who can lead you in the proper use of tonifying and dispersing herbs and foods. In addition, psychotherapy, spiritual counseling, acupuncture, and in some cases pharmaceutical and surgical interventions can also be employed to promote the return to balance when your systems have veered off course.

Other interventions such as diet and herbs, acupuncture, and Western medicine are all excellent tools and beyond the scope of this work. If you find you would like to pursue those avenues, I encourage you to seek out professional assistance. If you happen to be an herbalist, acupuncturist, or nutritionist, I encourage you to practice the arts of exercise, meditation, and touch therapy appearing in this book. I believe you will discover a powerful set of tools for enhanced healing understanding.

Practice with Touch Therapy

Touch therapy making use of the pathways of qi takes many forms, from self-administered tapping, brushing, and palpating techniques to a wide range of Asian bodywork therapy methods. The main common methods include various schools of shiatsu from Japan and styles of tuina from China. Basically, any manipulative therapy that works with the meridian channels in a specific and focused way can be considered

Asian bodywork therapy. Western massage therapy based on muscles and the physical systems of the body does not qualify as Asian bodywork therapy in that the standard Western massage therapy profession has little if any training in working with qi as it expresses itself in meridian organ network and elemental energy patterns.

When applying the touch techniques taught here, you are developing the fundamental skill sets required of a fully trained Asian bodywork therapist. This style of working the body is closer to physical therapy or chiropracty than it is to massage therapy and involves an education in channel energetics shared with the acupuncture profession. To learn a full hands-on therapeutic application of this healing method, live training with a qualified instructor is essential. For self-care as well as theoretical foundations, books and video are effective learning tools. The brushing and tapping routine offered below is an awesome personal cultivation tool and may be practiced safely and effectively. Give it a try and see for yourself the powerful benefits that can be discovered through activating the pathways of qi.

Brushing and Tapping—A Self-Care Routine

An excellent way to stimulate the qi in your body is through the simple practice of brushing and tapping. Brushing and tapping has the benefit of moving the channel toward equilibrium whether it is excess or deficient. The actual ability to assess states of deficiency and excess is a subtle skill that develops over time and usually with trained supervision. However, it is not necessary to be proficient at assessment prior to getting started. In fact, one could say that it is necessary to get started in order to become proficient. This is a very much a "learn by doing" system. As you gain experience, the ability to discern varying patterns and changes in your body, heartmind, and spirit will become easier.

Life is by its nature always predisposed toward balance. Just as spring faithfully follows winter each year and night and day consistently trade positions, so too our own natural state freely and easily alternates between yin and yang states of being as the movements of life demand. With brushing and tapping, we are becoming more deeply acquainted with the flow of the qi in the channels. In the process you learn and internalize the varying locations of each channel and the major points along the way. As you tap and brush, you feel the quality of the sensation at all given points and note that experience.

You may find some points are very sore, but with a slight change in rhythm or intensity of your brushing or tapping, the soreness will ease and the point will feel free and clear. After completing the entire sequence of brushing and tapping, you will have an overall sense of buzzing well-being. Enjoy the process of making yourself healthier and happier through encouraging your life energy to flow within your entire being.

Brushing the Channels

Brushing is generally performed before tapping; though it can be made to specifically follow each individual channel, it is often best to simply brush more generally over the yin and yang aspects of the body. Use your whole broad palm to accomplish the brushing and make gentle contact and off-the-body sweeping gestures over the surface. Begin with the yin aspect of one arm moving outward from chest to hand, brushing from the pectoralis, out toward the bicep and forearm to the open palm. Then turn your palm over and brush up the back of the forearm over the point of the elbow, up the tricep into the shoulder and up the side of the neck and ear to the face. Repeat on the other arm.

Once you've brushed to the face on the second arm, use both hands to brush over the top and sides of the head down to the neck and shoulders. Sweep down with your hands to the side ribs and allow your hands to spread wide so that they reach as far to the back as you can and also sweeps down the side of your torso. Sweep over the fullness of your buttocks and down the sides and backs of your thighs and legs. For this you will bend over to sweep down to the ankles, promoting flexibility through the forward bend.

Once at the feet, sweep your hands over to the bottoms of the feet and the inner ankle and sweep back up the inside of your leg and thigh to the groin area, the abdomen, and then into the chest. Begin again and sweep the entire body once more, shifting your hands slightly to get at any areas that may have been missed on the first pass. Repeat the entire sequence as many times as feels good and right to you.

The point of this brushing exercise is to gently sweep through your energy channels following the traditional direction of energy flow, invigorating and soothing your entire being. Practice differentiating the yin from the yang surfaces of the body, and internalize the classical direction of the energy flow. This is exactly as we learned the direction of energy in our journey through the one meridian flow. The yin arm channels flow from the torso out to your palms. The yang arm channels flow in from your hands to your face. The yang leg channels begin in the face and flow down and out through the feet, and the yin leg channels flow up from the bottoms of the feet to the torso.

As you become familiar with this flow, it will become second nature, and you will see that true to the yin and yang principles, the yin is of the earth and rises up from the bottoms of the feet to the torso and then from the torso moves up and out through the hands. The yang is of the heavens and it descends down through the finger tips and the top of the head to travel down the back and sides of the body to the feet. With this simple, elegant map, you can come to appreciate the exquisite position of being between the heavens and the earth. And you can begin to sense the balance involved in the joining of those powerful energies to create the body in which you live.

TAPPING THE MERIDIANS AND POINTS

The tapping routine is more vigorous than brushing. A certain attention should be paid to its invigorating nature. Where brushing is very gentle, tapping can sometimes be very strong. Be sensitive to your body's needs and don't overdo it just to prove something unless it is your nature to do so. If that's the case for you, note that and honor it, and be ready to deal with the consequences, whatever they may prove to be. Tapping is also more specific to channels and even points. To perform a Tapping routine, follow the one meridian flow outlined in chapter 1. Begin with Lung 1 and follow the sequence all the way through to Liver 14. Use the images of meridian and point locations and function covered in chapters 2 through 7 to deepen your overall practice.

Tapping the entire circuit of the body will take about five to ten minutes or more. Be sure to allow adequate time to complete the entire sequence. If you should get distracted in the middle, don't worry, you won't do any damage with this method. Simply take note of where you left off, or at what point you became distracted. Then pick up from where you left off, or simply restart from the beginning. If you find that over the course of a week's practice you continue to get distracted at the same point, then it is likely that you are getting a message about that particular channel being neglected or avoided.

As you tap through the sequence, allow yourself to give particular attention to points near the joints and to any point that calls attention to itself through sensitivity either pleasurable or uncomfortable. The points at the joints are all major points in the system and as such have a certain efficacy and preeminence in our work. Points that demonstrate peculiar reactions to the contact are communicating something of note. As particular points stand out among all the rest as having significantly different response to the contact, you can consult the list of major points to get some clue about which function may be asking for more attention.

Of course, knowing which channel a sensation is on is a starting place for interpreting the messages your body is sending you. Next would be the actual specific point itself. There is a great wealth of information here in this book, and in the vast literature available on Chinese medicine you can find information on the working functions of each and every point on the body. However, I encourage you not to simply take the information in the charts and books as gospel. Make sure to apply your own personal experience and consideration as the last word. There are many possible interpretations of what sensitivity at any given point could mean. And the most important interpretation is the one you derive from your own personal experience. You, after all, have lived in your body your entire life, and you are the only one in possession of the most intimate and detailed information on what your body might be telling you with any given sensation.

That said, the primary method for tapping is to form your fingers into what is known as the crane's beak. This is a hand position in which the thumb and four fingers are all drawn together. You then proceed to tap in a rhythmic fashion on your body, following the pathways of the energy channels and taking time at each point along the way. Trust your intuitive sense of how long and how hard to tap on each point. It is not important that the crane's beak be held tightly together, in fact a loose wrist action and loose fingers produces the best result. On various points in some sections of the body, you'll want to change from the crane's beak to the karate chop or the light fist. Experiment with these various hand positions for the tapping hand.

Start at Lung on one side; it doesn't matter which. Tap the channel from Lung 1 to 11. Turn the arm being tapped and start on the Large Intestine, tapping from 1 to 20. As you tap into the face, be particularly light with your finger tapping. After completing Large Intestine on the first side, move to Lung on the second side and then Large Intestine as well. End at Large Intestine 20 in the face.

Next move to Stomach meridian in the face, lightly tapping with both hands on both sides at the same time. Tap from 1 to 8, and then drop down to tap 9 in the neck and on down through the torso to 30 at the pubic bone. Lighten up over the breast tissue, and remember the channels narrows to two inches off centerline as you move down the abdomen. After Stomach 30, tap across the inguinal ligaments out to Stomach 31 at the top of the vastus lateralis muscle in the thigh. Here switch to a light fist and give the muscle a good pounding as you follow the channel all the way down the thigh across the knee and along the tibialis anterior, the shin muscle. Switch back to crane's beak in the top of the foot, ending with Stomach 45 in the second toe.

After completing Stomach switch over with crane's beak finger taps to follow the Spleen channel up from Spleen 1 in the big toe to Spleen 9 at the knee. In the thigh, switch back to a light fist and continue up to the inguinal ligaments. Here you'll want to switch back to the crane's beak as you cross the sensitive inguinal triangle and follow the channel up through the abdomen to the breast tissue, tailing down to its completion at Spleen 21. It's tricky to tap Spleen 21 on both sides at the same time. You may want to try crossing your hands over to tap with the crane's beak from the opposite side of the body, and do one side at a time. Spleen 21 is a very influential point and you'll want to make sure to give it a good tapping out.

Next we are back at the arms and we move on through the one meridian flow to Heart and Small Intestine. Again you'll need to do one side at a time. You'll find that crane's beak works well for Heart, but Small Intestine is a little tricky. Try using karate chop, or even Large Intestine 4 as the contact point for tapping out Small Intestine from 1 through 9. For Small Intestine 10 and 11 in the shoulder blade, use an open fingered slapping action to get down into the area of the infraspinous fossa. You'll revert to crane's beak for Small Intestine 12 through in the top of the shoulder and neck to 18 and 19 in the face.

After tapping Heart and Small Intestine on one side, switch over and tap out the same lines and points on the other side. Completing at Small Intestine 19, shift over to tapping both sides simultaneously again as you pick up Bladder 1 through 4 in the forehead with crane's beak. Switch to the knuckles of a loose fist as you tap over the top of the head from 4 to 10. Use fingertips for 11, and reach back as far as you can between your shoulder blades to try and reach Bladder 12 and maybe 13. There's an area in your back between the shoulder blades that you'll probably need to accept that you just can't reach unless you have extremely flexible shoulders. Once you've reached down as far as you can from above, switch your arms around and use the back of your fist as high up the back as you can reach, and then continue to tap on down the rest of the Bladder channel down to the sacrum and buttocks.

Now turn your tapping hands and use the front of the loose fist for the sacrum, buttocks, and thigh and calf points, switching to crane's beak for the points of the ankle and foot. End up with a nice tapping along the outer edge of the foot to Bladder 67.

To tap out the Kidney meridian, you have to contort your body somewhat into a wide-legged squat position, but not too wide and not too deep. You'll find just the right position for yourself as you practice. Invert the foot, rolling up on to the outer edges and exposing points Kidney 1 and 2 to your finger tips. As you shift into the inner ankle points Kidney 3 through 6, relax the inversion of your feet but keep the feet turned out, so that you can directly tap on Kidney 6 through 10 in the inner calf. Continue the turn out as you tap up the channel from the knee to the groin, and crossing the groin gently arrive at the pubic bone and tap with your crane's beak up the Kidney channel just a half-inch off centerline in the abdomen and two inches off centerline in the chest, all the way to Kidney 27. It may be tender through the chest points, so modulate your intensity as needed. At the same time, realize this is an essential vital energy boosting technique, so don't be shy.

Pericardium channel is next and as you return to the arms, you'll again have to do one side at a time. Choose either side to start, it makes no difference. Crane's beak works best for the Pericardium from just outside the nipple and moving up the anterior deltoid and out into the bicep. After the bicep, try a loose fist in the forearm. That can be deeply invigorating. Gage your own level of need and find the quality of stimulation that is most effective for you.

As you cross over the palm and then turn the arm to present Triple Warmer, you may find that you naturally are drawn to using a loose fist to tap out the Triple Warmer meridian back up the arm, over the shoulder and into the neck. The shoulder points of Triple Warmer often present as particularly appreciative of a good solid pounding. Go ahead, drop the weight of the world from your shoulders and let them have it! Continuing when you are ready, the crane's beak once more works well for the Triple Warmer points around the ear. As you cross the temple, however, shift to using gentle finger tapping once more. Repeat Pericardium and Triple Warmer on the second arm.

After completing the second arm, tap Triple Warmer 23 on both sides at the same time with gentle finger tapping. Drop a half-inch down to Gall Bladder 1 and follow the channel to tap each of the points 1 through 14. As you tap 15 through 20, switch to the knuckles of the light fist once more. The side of the skull can really respond to this knocking. I always get the image of knocking some sense into my head. But remember, in gentleness there is great strength, so don't overdo it.

Gall Bladder 20 through 29 respond really well to crane's beak and various modifications of a loose finger tapping. Be sure to circuit back and forth along the channel and stimulate each and every point along the way. Use the images from chapter 1 as a guide until you commit the pathways to memory. Once you arrive at GB 30 in the buttocks, make a light fist again and tap down the channel along the side of the leg from 30 to 40 at the ankle. In the foot, use crane's beak to finish the flow into the fourth toe.

Continue to use finger tips as you pick up Liver in the big toe and tap it up to the ankle. Try light knuckles on the lower shin Liver 5 and 6, and then karate chop on the calf and inner thigh to stimulate Liver 7 through 11. Finger tap once more across the inguinal ligaments and into the abdominals out to the tip of the eleventh floating rib where you find Liver 13. Finally, tap up to Liver 14, the Gate of the Cycle in the sixth intercostal space just below the breast tissue. Complete by reconnecting to Lung 1 once more, and then relax.

Congratulations! You've just completed a full tapping out of the channel system. Take a moment to appreciate all the many sensations of circulation and life energy stimulation that result from this delicious exercise. Breath a few deep breaths and shower your body with infinite love and gratitude. You have just honored your body as the vessel of your being. Hold on to the preciousness of who you are.

As you practice this exercise over time and become more proficient in your knowledge of channel and point location, you can add in awareness of the functions of each channel and even individual points along the way as you tap through the body. This is truly a powerful and effective tool for enhancing whole body health and awareness. Take it to the next level. Enjoy your life and your body—it's the only one you've got.

If you find that you really want to up the ante on bringing this routine effectively into your daily life, take a moment to write down a few thoughts about which points and lines were most sensitive. Track this quality of sensation day by day and watch it change.

Deepen your practice by studying the meridian channels and point names, and commit them to memory. Begin to see how the sensitivities you find in various points correlates to the functions of the meridian channels described in chapters 2 through 7. In this way you can begin to truly come to know yourself and your energy flows in a deeply profound and useful way.

Remember to keep studying. In the next chapters, we're going to dive deeper into the study of life and self that presents itself to us through the pathways of qi.

Chapter 9

Meridian Energy Flow, Personality and the Five Elements

The study of self, self-expression, and character is perhaps one of the most compelling studies of humanity. How is it that we are all human and yet express ourselves and our character is such unique and various ways? How is that we come to be who we are, and come to know ever more deeply who we are as we progress through life? In this chapter, let's take the awareness of meridians and the effects of qi energy even deeper with the study of constitution, temperament and personality through contemplations and meditations on the energy channels.

Over the years I have taught the following material many, many of times to hundreds of people. It is always deeply engaging and fascinating. As you read through what I share with you here, I encourage you to begin to realize that it is actually the distribution of your qi energy in various strengths and levels throughout your meridian system that makes you who you are. And the good news is that by working with the qi energy directly in your meridians channels, you can have a profound influence on who you are, the things you do or do not like about yourself, and how you show up in the world. You can use the information I give you here to re-shape your life so that you become more and more the person that you were meant to be in this life.

We all go through life trying to figure out in one way or another who we are and what we are here for. Family, culture, and society as well as pre-endowed characteristics of gender, ethnicity, shape, and size deeply influence our sense of self. And the various facets of our constitution, Temperament and personality can ultimately be seen as expressions of the energy of our meridian channels, both in what we are endowed with at birth, and what we choose to cultivate and develop over the course of our life time. Take this work to heart, and discover how you can put the pathways of qi to work for you in being the best you can be.

Functions of the Five Elements and the Twelve Regular Channels in Developing Personality

Each of the meridian channels has an influence over a wide range of human functions. By understanding the unique expressions of each, we come to understand that who we are. Every aspect of our being is shaped and influenced by the quality and quantity of energy in any given channel.

There are many systems of personality being promoted and taught in the world today, the enneagram, astrological signs, archetypes, and so on—all of these systems are similar in scope to the meridian personality system we will be exploring here, offered so you can have a deeper idea of how the meridian energies of life affect the person you are and the way you appear in the world. This in turn will deepen your practice of touch and meridian movements to help you discover deeper and deeper levels of self-realization.

Equipping yourself with this powerful system for self-reflection you can position yourself for tremendous personal growth. When I first learned this system, certain unruly aspects of my own character came into view.

The knowledge I gained here helped me to learn to moderate those aspects and develop parts of myself that had long been neglected.

This is the personality system used in the therapeutic application of HeartMind Shiatsu. It is directly correlated to the pathways of qi at the core of the practice of HeartMind Shiatsu and Meridian Gesture Qigong and gives us a powerful set of tools for understanding the meridian energy flows and the various manifestations of excess and deficient energy patterns.

The meridian personalities described here are drawn from the works of the French acupuncturist and clinician Yves Requena with supportive understandings from the five element understanding of acupuncturists Harriet Beinfield and Efrem Korngold. I have also brought in the insightful correlations of acupuncturist and psychiatrist Leon Hammer, the Master Japanese Shiatsu Therapist Shizuto Masunaga, as well as my own clinical and classroom experiences to bring this model into its current form.

The works of Requena, Beinfield, Korngold, Hammer, and Masunaga are all referenced in the bibliography, and you can find out more about each of these outstanding clinicians and their contribution to the field by acquiring their written works referenced there.

At the outset it is important to note that this work with human expressions of personality is being correlated to Traditional Chinese Medicine. The descriptions of such an understanding of the five elements and the twelve meridians and their relationship to personality given here are not drawn directly from ancient sources. Rather, some keen insights from Western psychology are overlaid on the Chinese channel system. Many scholars call this "forcing" and refute its efficacy on grounds that it is not thoroughly grounded in classical referents. Personally, I find it is important to acknowledge such comment and welcome it here as well. Such critical attention is crucial to the dialogue amongst professionals.

At any rate, it is extremely important to read any such material with a skeptical and critical eye. At the same time, direct clinical experience and application in the modern Western world is essential to maintaining the vibrancy of the model for Western sensibilities. With that in mind, let's explore the system of personality types that I work from in the HeartMind Shiatsu model.

Constitution, Temperament, and Personality

To begin, it is important to note, as Leon Hammer states so eloquently, that "stereotyping someone is ultimately an abhorrent and dehumanizing process."[4] No one is a pure type; it is a form of injustice to reduce people to a given category or type. "However," he goes on, "it is clinically useful." In addition, I have found, and my colleagues agree, that even in applying this personality model no one actually appears as a pure type, but rather they show up as a composite of personality traits. Each of us actually has a range of energetic possibilities. In some cases, we are strong in one aspect but weak in others, but this does not mean that we cannot adapt and change given circumstances and proper skilled practice.

It is also important here to make a distinction between constitution, temperament and personality as I use the terms here. Generally, constitutional and temperamental factors are more directly attributed to the influence of the five elements and are present from birth. In Chinese, the word *xing* is translated as both as "constitution" and "temperament" and refers to enduring characteristics of a human being. What I'm interested in here are the more fluid aspects of human character that grow and develop over time. For the purposes of this discussion, I will use the word "personality," referring to the more changeable and variable characteristics of our being with this term, granting us the possibility for a range of responses in any given situation.

These aspects of being are more directly related to meridian differentiation and have a certain degree of adaptability over the course of a lifetime due to conditioning and environmental factors. As to constitu-

---

4   Hammer, L. *Dragon Rises, Redbird Flies,* Easton Press, Seattle, 2005, p48.

tion, Beinfield, and Korngold maintain that your elemental type is "like your blood type."[5] You are born of a certain elemental constitution that will be your constitutional bias for life. I have found no significant evidence to the contrary. But at the level of personality as I am defining it here, there is a greater range of flexibility and the possibility for change over the course of time and circumstance. These constitutional archetypes are central to the character of any given person, and even these cursory descriptions may have already set off bells of recognition in your mind about your own way of being in the world or someone you know. As constitutional factors, they comprise the base note of each individual's view of and contribution to life. As we proceed into the more detailed discussion of temperament and personality, we will certainly see these elemental characteristics reflected in each.

The constitutional types as outlined by Beinfield and Korngold are as follows: The Fire element creates the Wizard. These are the persons of great personal dynamism who can amaze and transform situations and lives through their powerful and charismatic Fire element affinities. The Earth element in abundance yields the archetype of the Peacemaker. Ever interested in the well-being and sustenance of all, the Earth element abhors injustice and therefore lends itself to the efforts of making peace in the world. The Metal element gives us the Alchemist. This persona has the ability to take base metals and transform them into gold. Concerned with propriety, etiquette, and morality, the Metal element grants the power to refine and mature to perfection. The Water element shapes the Philosopher. Concerned with the deeper pondering of life and death, the Water element runs deep, and its strong presence in a person's energy field will yield the deep thinking and reflective depths of the philosopher. Finally, the Wood element gives us the Pioneer. Ever concerned with growth and

---

5   Beinfeld, H and Korngold, E, *Between Heaven and Earth*, Ballantine Books, New York, 1991, p134.

change and forging forward into new ground, the Wood element brings forth the pioneering spirit in the individual, destined to lead the way and chart the course forward for all of humanity.

These constitutional archetypes are central to the character of any given person, and even these cursory descriptions may have already set off alarm bells of recognition in your mind either about your own way of being in the world or someone you know. As constitutional factors they make up the base note of each individual's view of and contribution to life. As we proceed into the more detailed discussion of personality, we will certainly see these elemental characteristics reflected in each.

As we engage in the discussion of personality as compared to constitution, we will inevitably arrive at an important differentiation between the five element and meridian influences. To set the stage for that discussion it is important to see that elements have a wide range of governance, each having both yin and yang manifestations. When we expand our discussion to the more varied descriptions of personality we expand out in to the twelve regular meridian channels each of which is either yin or yang. This is an important distinction, for as we will see below, yin and yang and the various levels and qualities of the yin and yang have a strong bearing on personality.

The primary model I use here for differentiating the major aspects of personality is drawn from a body of Western psychology Requena masterfully reconciled to match the Chinese channel system. Central to this discussion is the work of "schools of objective experimental and quantitative psychology that include comparative and pathological psychology. Gaston Berger, a French researcher and protégé of Le Senne developed character types that were originally introduced by the Dutch school of Heymans and Wiersma."[6] This character system yielded eight

---

6   Requena, Yves, *Character and Health: The Relationship of Acupuncture and Psychology,* Brookline, MA, Paradigm Publications, 1989, p41.

"temperament types." Requena ingeniously grafted these eight "temperament types" onto the energetics of the twelve regular channels. Following is a description of the methodology and thinking behind the definition of each type and its correlation to the meridian channels. And my invitation and discovery is to let go of thinking of these types as rigid enduring characteristics of constitution and temperament, and allow them to be the more malleable and adaptable characteristics of personality, growth and possibility.

Let's explore how these various aspects of personality can be discovered and discerned. To arrive at eight distinct character types, Berger created "a method for determining the degree to which emotivity, activity, and resonance were expressed in an individual."[7] Each of these aspects of personal expression can be seen upon a continuum. Emotivity ranges from Emotional to Non-emotional, Activity ranges form Active to Inactive, and Resonance ranges from Primary to Secondary.

The first two aspects of Emotivity and Activity are relatively self evident, but the last quality of Resonance needs some discussion. Resonance is related to one's reaction time to any given situation. Someone who is governed by primary influences is one who acts rashly and on impulse without much (if any) forethought. A secondary expression is descriptive of one who acts prudently and cautiously with meditative consideration. Given that this language seems to be a bit like jargon for academics, I have translated the terms "Primary" and "Secondary" into "Spontaneous" and "Meditative" respectively.

Now when we take these three qualities and their manifestations at the ends of their continuum and combine them into all possible combinations we get eight distinct expressions of character as follows:

---

7   Requena, Yves, *Character and Health: The Relationship of Acupuncture and Psychology,* Brookline, MA, Paradigm Publications, 1989, p42.

1. Active, Emotive, Spontaneous

2. Active, Emotive, Meditative

3. Active, Non-Emotive, Spontaneous

4. Active, Non-Emotive, Meditative

5. Non-Active, Emotive, Spontaneous

6. Non-Active, Emotive, Meditative

7. Non-Active, Non-Emotive, Spontaneous

8. Non-Active, Non-Emotive, Meditative

To understand these eight characterizations more fully, imagine 1 as a person who takes action, imbues their action with emotional intensity or passion, and acts in a spontaneous fashion. Contrast this person with person 2, who takes action, imbues their action with passion, yet thinks twice before acting. Carry this forward for each of the eight characterizations and you will begin to see the shadings of character that manifest from one type to the next.

Now we graft these eight characteristics onto the meridian channel system with some creative imagination and scholarship. The first stop along the way is to see which of the expressive qualities relates to which meridian or elemental energy. Right away we determine that active and non-active is expressive of yang and yin, yin being non-active, yang being active. Therefore, all the Active-type personality characteristics are related to yang channels, and the Non-Active characteristics are related to yin channels. Emotivity is a quality granted to the Fire element. Think of the warmth and flash of emotional expression and you can see how Fire is the natural element governing this characteristic. Spontaneity is a factor descriptive of the Earth, Wood and supplemental Fire elements. Each of these elements govern the ability to act quickly and get the job at hand accomplished without a great deal of second guessing. Finally, meditative is a quality ascribed to Metal, Water, and absolute Fire. These elements are tasked with taking the long view, being able to step back from immediate engagement, and then support a well-thought out approach to a given situation.[8]

Knowing which expressive quality is granted by the elements and which by an attribute of the six divisions of yin and yang gives us the formula we need to correlate these aspects of personality to the meridians. To do so, we simply need to look at the ways in which the meridians are paired.

In five element pairings there are two meridians in each element, one yang and one yin. In the six divisions of yin and yang, the channels are paired up based on their level of yin or yang. We explored these levels earlier; Tai Yang, Yang Ming, and Shao Yang, and Tai Yin, Jue Yin, and Shao Yin. We can translate these as "most Yang", "middle Yang," and "least Yang", and "most Yin", "middle Yin," and "least Yin". The six divisions give us the following pairings.

Tai Yang includes the yang channels of absolute Fire and Water, the Small Intestine, and the Bladder. These are the yang channels of the "back" body.

Yang Ming includes the yang channels of Earth and Metal and the Stomach and the Large Intestine. These are the yang channels of the "front" body.

Shao Yang includes the yang channels of supplemental Fire and Wood and the Triple Warmer and the Gall Bladder. These are the yang channels of the "side" body.

Tai Yin includes the yin channels of Earth and Metal and the Spleen/Pancreas and the Lungs. These are the yin channels of the "front" body.

Jue Yin includes the yin channels of Supplemental Fire and Wood, the Pericardium and the Liver. These are the channels of the "side" body.

Shao Yin includes the yin channels of absolute Fire and Water and the Heart and the Kidneys. These are the yin channels of the "back" body.

---

8   Requena, Yves, *Character and Health: The Relationship of Acupuncture and Psychology,* Brookline, MA, Paradigm Publications, 1989, p45–50.

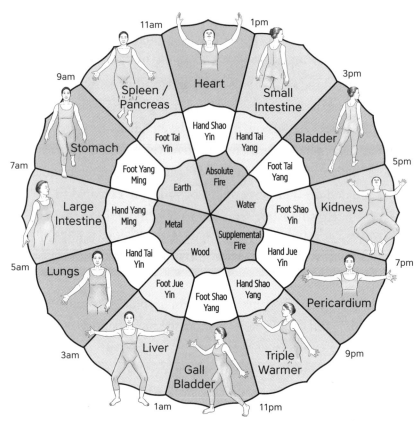

Figure 15: This wheel shows the six yin and six yang channels
and their corresponding element, meridian, and time.

With these pairings we now take the eight aspects of personality and
graft them into place.

The Tai Yang pair is a combination of absolute Fire and Water. It is
Active because it is yang, Emotive because of the presence of absolute
Fire, and Meditative because Water and absolute Fire both share this
characteristic.

The Shao Yang pair is a combination of supplemental Fire and Wood.
It is Active because it is yang, Emotive because of the presence of Supple-

mental Fire, and Spontaneous because supplemental Fire and Wood both lend spontaneity to the character.

The Yang Ming pair includes both Earth and Metal. It is Active because it is yang and non-emotive because Earth and Metal are both Non-emotive. But there is a split that shows up here between Stomach and Large Intestine—because Earth is Spontaneous and Metal is Meditative, we end up with two distinct character types in the Yang Ming: Yang Ming Earth and Yang Ming Metal.

The Tai Yin pairing also includes both Earth and Metal. And now because it is yin, we see that it is Non-active. It is Non-Emotive because Earth and Metal both lend non-emotivity to the character, and here there is another split of the pair because Earth is spontaneous and Metal is Meditative. So we have the Tai Yin Earth and the Tai Yin Metal personality characteristics.

The Jue Yin pair is made up of Supplemental Fire and Wood. It is a Non-Active type because it is yin, Emotive because of the influence of Supplemental Fire on the pair, and Spontaneous as both Supplemental Fire and Wood lend spontaneity to the character.

The Shao Yin pair consists of both Absolute Fire and Water. Again, this pairing lends to the idea of being Non-Active because it is yin. Emotive because of the presence of Absolute Fire in the pair, and Meditative due to the presence of Water and Absolute Fire in the pair.

Of course it is laborious to draw this all out each and every time we discuss a personality characteristic, so fortunately there are descriptive adjectives that go with each type. The Tai Yang earns itself the distinction of Passionate, for the Tai Yang energy animates acts of passion. Shao Yang holds sway over Enthusiastic types, for their particular brand of behavior is marked by "enthusiastic and vigorous" displays. The Yang Ming Earth gains the distinction of Robust-Sanguine, for its fine animation of the appetite that is ruled by the Stomach. Like Seymour the man-eating plant in *Little Shop of Horrors,* the personality governed by Stomach is happy to say "Feed Me! You look chunky!"[9] And Yang Ming Metal animates the Precise-Phlegmatic aspect of our character, being ever concerned with the details and the rules of the game of life.

As we move into the Yin aspect of our being, we find the softer side of human personality. These tend to be the types that are less dominant in society, more reclusive and introspective. To begin, the Tai Yin Earth, Spleen/Pancreas quality grabs the title of Amorphous/Chameleon. The Spleen/Pancreas with its penchant for sweetness and pleasure assists us in knowing how to blend in with any crowd. The Tai Yin Metal, Lung quality governs the Apathetic/Aloof aspects of our nature, the aspects which hold themselves apart, seeing all clearly yet participating in none. The Jue Yin, Liver and Pericardium energy level expresses itself as Sensitive-Dramatic, having strong emotions, moody reactions, and spontaneous "flutterings." And finally the Shao Yin, Heart and Kidney captures the expression of our Sentimental nature, ever expressive of our deep yearning for intimacy and the underlying connections with life and death, vitality, and introversion.

As we explore each of these aspects of personality, we see snapshots of ourselves and people we know. Keep in mind, however, the cautionary note sounded by Leon Hammer—we must beware not to dehumanize anyone with typology. And yet we may use the information clinically, finding it useful in looking at the patterns of personal expression and particularly how these relate to the relative balance of qi energy in the meridian pathways.

For example, if you find that you are too sensitive and dramatic (Jue Yin), you may indulge the development of your passionate Tai Yang nature to attain some balance. You do this by holding the qi energy of Liver and Pericardium in check while increasing the amount of energy in your Small Intestine and Bladder. If you find you are too lusty and sanguine

---

9 Griffith, Charles B. *Little Shop of Horrors*, FilmGroup, Inc, 1960.

(Yang Ming Earth), you may need to develop your sentimental Shao Yin aspects for greater depth and scope in your dealings with others. Here you curtail the unruly rumblings and compulsions of your Stomach and get quiet and inward with the true depths of your being as expressed through Heart and Kidney. If your enthusiastic Shao Yang nature has run like a bull through a china shop, it may be time to call upon the precise-phlegmatic Yang Ming Metal aspects of your demeanor and come into the bright, white light of accountability. In short, constrain your Gall Bladder and bring in the attention to detail and care that is granted to you by the power of qi in the Large Intestine.

These are just a few examples of how you might use your sense of meridian qi flowing through your channels to have an influence over the way you show up in the world. The combinations and interactions of the meridian energies are infinite. Studying them each separately and then discovering how they combine and work together in unique and powerful ways in each person gives us a powerful tool for growth, development and ultimately true self-realization.

It is important to note that we have all twelve meridian channels working within our system. So by extension, we all have all the energetic aspects of personality within us as well. Sometimes we are deficient in one and excess in another. Through directed and well crafted tonification and sedation we can work to achieve greater balance and harmony. Any of the aspects of our personality, if too strong or too weak can wreak havoc on our sense of balance in the world. And by the same token, each has a steady, healthy, balanced expression, for each has its task to perform. To have a full range of expression of all the channels is to have a full and satisfying life. And to recognize where we are weak and where we are strong gives us the chance to move and change and adapt to our circumstances leading to our highest cultivation and optimal health.

Short Listing of Personality Traits

Following are general short lists of personality traits that I have derived from a combination of sources. These exist within the realm of the "conditioned layer of health" discussed in chapter 1. This is the level of cultivation most closely related to the HeartMind and all its permutations and manifestations in thoughts, feelings, habits, attitudes, and beliefs. I invite you to pour over them and discover for yourself how the qualities listed correlate to the criteria of Active/Inactive, Emotive/Non-emotive and Spontaneous/Meditative that are hallmarks of individual personality.

Challenge your understanding to begin to see these attributes as being true to the understanding of the meridian channel functions explored in chapters 2 through 7. And finally, see how the various surface areas of the body, through which the meridians flow, offer a reflection of these facets of personality. This is truly learning to read body language in its many intricate and sophisticated, and often unconscious expressions.

Tai Yang Traits

Key Traits of the Small Intestine Hand Tai Yang: Passionate personality, seeks accomplishment, discerning, higher judgment, superior, ambitious, presumptuous, arrogant

Key Traits of the Bladder Foot Tai Yang: Passionate personality, most likely to succeed, brilliant, deep, driven toward goals, self-sacrificing, domineering, hypersensitive, grandiose

Yang Ming Traits

Key Traits of the Large Intestine Hand Yang Ming: Precise-Phlegmatic personality, keeper of the rules, reliable, anal retentive, perfectionist, persnickety, duty–bound, great sense of humor

Key Traits of the Stomach Foot Yang Ming: Lusty-Sanguine personality, ruled by appetite, opportunist, initiator, superficial, socially adept, born leader, ends justify means

Shao Yang Traits

Key Traits of the Triple Warmer Hand Shao Yang: Enthusiastic personality, protector of the body, sharer of warmth, can also give the cold shoulder, the betrayer and betrayed, exuberant, broad shouldered, hard working, optimist

Key HeartMind Traits of the Gall Bladder Foot Shao Yang: Enthusiastic personality, defender of the law, hyper-responsible, self-important, pretentious, assertive-aggressive, all sinew, hyperactive, party animal

Tai Yin Traits

Key HeartMind Traits of the Lung Hand Tai Yin: Aloof personality, house of the qi essence, polite, cautious, takes in qi energy, sighing, choking, breathing, thick skinned, ethical, creature of habit.

Key HeartMind Traits of the Spleen Foot Tai Yin: Amorphous-Chameleon personality, house of the Moisture essence, pleasure driven, sweet toothed, soft, comfortable, nourisher, nurturer, calm, humble, happy-go-lucky

Jue Yin Traits

Key Traits of the Pericardium Hand Jue Yin: Nervous-Dramatic personality, protector of the Spirit essence, emotional, moody, warm, compassionate, crimes of passion, circulation issues, anxious, erratic, needy

Key Traits of the Liver Foot Jue Yin: Nervous-Dramatic personality, house of the Blood essence, visionary planner, chief executive, addict, swears and curses, demonstrated anger and control, emotionally volatile or smooth as silk
Shao Yin Traits

Key Traits of the Heart Hand Shao Yin: Sentimental personality, house of the Spirit essence, sees the high truth, great interpreter, thrives in intimacy, rhythm master, hyper-emotive, joyful, excitable

Key Traits of the Kidney Foot Shao Yin: Sentimental personality, house of the Vital essence, strong constitution, introverted, dislikes crowds, strong, weak or balanced libido, hypersensitive, fearful, withdrawn

Practice with Meditation

Now it's time to put all this contemplation to work in deepening self-realization through these specially crafted elemental meditations. I developed the meditations to allow you to have a deep experience in your body of the ways in which the primal elemental energies manifest in your daily life. By more fully understanding each of these qualities, you come into possession of a deeper self-knowing and are able to better understand why certain things happen or don't happen in your world. With practice, you can begin to slowly shift your experience in life to get more of the things you want, and reduce the things you do not want. Allow these meditations to work their magic, and open your eyes to a whole new world of self-understanding.

A Six-Step Process to Greater Self-Realization

As we have been studying and discovering through our study of the pathways of qi, life energy runs through the body along specific channels, which animate and govern all of our life functions. The flow of this energy is much like the flow of energy in nature that moves the earth through the seasons of the year. The pathways can be seen running through the body, one leading to the other in an endless ongoing circulation of energy. The order in which the meridians and their governing elemental influences are sequenced follows the energy demands of an average daily life in a logical pattern. In addition, the meditations upon the elements which follow in the order of the daily cycle of energy flow constitute a thorough and profound energetic process to greater self-realization.

The meditations which follow will take you on just this journey. Follow them in this order, each one building upon the previous. You will begin at the surface with Metal, move deeper in with Earth, deeper still with absolute Fire and Water, and then begin your journey back out with supplemental Fire and finally Wood. Take your time; do them all at once in an hour or two, once a day for six days, or once a week for six weeks. Allow yourself time to walk into each level of your being with each meditation and see your whole being through this powerful lens.

An Overview of Elemental Meditations and the Practice of Being Fully Alive

Go through the sequence of the six meditations of the daily cycle of energy flow and consider how the cycle takes you from the superficial to the deep and back to the surface again. You'll go from acknowledging your boundaries, to seeing what you are made of, to giving yourself permission to hold yourself precious and protect and defend yourself.

Go through the meditations as often as you wish to fortify your self-understanding and to develop any areas in your being that are deficient and soften any aspects which appear to be excessive. Go over the following summary of the elements in the daily cycle and take time to note your perception of your strengths and weaknesses at this time in your life.

Metal: Perhaps you don't have a sense of your own boundaries and too often you find yourself relinquishing any right to your own point of view. Or perhaps your boundaries are too rigid allowing for no influence whatsoever from the outside. This relates to Metal because of the nature of boundaries and connections. It expressed through the body in the Lung and Large Intestine meridians. By following this meditation, you will strengthen your sense of self.

Earth: Are you aware of what truly nourishes you in your life and do you allow yourself to receive it, or do you push it away? Do you deserve to be nourished? If not, you are starving. If so, you are thriving. In some cases, you may be stuffing yourself with things that don't truly nourish you; though they fill you up, the feeling is temporary and in the end meaningless.

Fire (absolute): Who are you? Truly…what makes you tick? What do you believe in? What is your highest truth? If you are uncertain and wavering in your own viewpoint, you are deficient in this area. If you are way too sure of yourself, you may be just a bit overzealous and burning yourself out.

Water: What are your deepest innermost feelings of life and death? Do you cherish life or is it tedious? Do you even have any deep feelings about it, or are you just going along to get along? Are you driven to move forward in life, or would you rather just sit and watch the world go by?

Fire (supplemental): Are you prepared for life and all it sends your way? Does life warm you up, and surround you with feelings of safety and contentment, or are you always on your guard, waiting for the other shoe to drop? How much energy do you put into locked doors, safety deposit boxes, and security systems? Are you excessively overprotected and alone in the world? Or do you mingle in good company and experience the warmth of human contact? Do you consider yourself precious?

Wood: Do you know how to stand your ground and stick to your guns through thick and thin? Or are you a fart in the wind, a leaf on a lake?

STEP ONE: YOUR PERSONAL BOUNDARIES—JOURNEY INTO METAL

The Lung and Large Intestine are the representatives of the Metal element in the body. Metal is all that is precious. It is structure, interconnection and interconnectivity, the intricate webbing of life that stretches between all things.

Lie down in a comfortable position and focus inward on your breath. Watch the breath go in and out of your body. As much as you can, don't try to control your breath, simply get out of the way and watch the phenomenon of breathing. The body/mind knows how to do this without your knowledge or consent. Though it may be difficult it is possible to observe without controlling. Once you have achieved this state, you will experience a sense of awe and wonder at the process of life.

Rest in that sense of awe for a moment, and then turn your mind to consider your personal boundary, the very edges of yourself, where you end and the rest of the world begins. See yourself as a sovereign nation and take a moment to place yourself in the role of the customs official, the border patrol of your own nation.

Start at the physical level. See the size and shape of your body-nation. Feel your weight as it presses into the floor. Sense the air as it flows around your body. Feel the edges of your physical being. In this state of awareness, consider your physical abilities, how much weight you can lift, how fast you can run, how high you can jump. Feel the edges, the limits of your physical abilities. Breathe in and breathe out, and slowly let that go as you return to simply being present.

Turn your attention now to the mental level of your being. Consider your thoughts and the limits of your intellect. What stimulates your mind? What do you find boring? What goes over your head?

How widely have you read? At what level of language do you converse? What is your IQ? Recall a mind teaser puzzle, are you quick to figure it out, or does it take you a great deal of time? Are you unable to figure them out? What are the edges of your mind? Breathe in and breathe out and ponder the limits of your intellect, and slowly let that go as you return to simply being present.

Now consider your emotional boundaries. How sensitive are you? Do you cry easily? How long was it since you last laughed out loud? Blew your top? Trembled and hid beneath the covers? What sets you off emotionally? Where is your emotional boundary? Where is that line between where your experience of the world spills over into the feelings that you have about the world? Consider your emotional boundaries, when, where, and how you allow your emotions to be acknowledged and expressed. Take your time. Breathe in and out and let that go as you return to simply being present.

Now consider your spiritual being. How big is your spirit, how vast? Where is the edge where your spirit meets the spirit of another, with the great spirit of all that is? Let yourself feel this edge if you can find it, or allow yourself to drift off into a sense of oneness with all that is allowing your boundaries to dissolve. Feel yourself floating on waves of universal life energy, rising and falling smoothly and effortlessly. Then let that go too and return to your breath.

Once more feel your body lying on the floor and recognize your being as a sovereign nation. See yourself in the role of minister of trade. As a human being you are not separate and autonomous, but rather you rely on a certain level of exchange with all that is around you in order to survive. Your Metal element is like the customs house agent, and the minister of trade that monitors everything that comes into you from outside and everything you give out to the world from inside yourself.

Do you have a trade deficit, or surplus? How is the balance of trade between your friends and family and the rest of the world? Breathe in and breathe out, and find yourself fully present to the moment right where you are, once more witnessing the miracle of breath without need to alter its course or judge its quality. Simply observe, without judgment, a sovereign being in the sovereign land of your own body, heartmind, and spirit.

Slowly come out of the meditation and take time to discuss your experience with a friend, make notes in your journal, or create a work of art that depicts your own personal boundaries.

STEP TWO: WHAT ARE YOU HUNGRY FOR?— JOURNEY INTO EARTH

Here we are focusing on the Stomach meridian and Spleen meridian, which are the representatives of the Earth element in the body and heart-mind. They are the organ networks through which nourishment comes into our being. You can see this correlation with the earth when you think of the deep rich soil and foundation of our home planet that provides for our every need in life.

Turn inward once more, lying on your stomach this time. Breathe down and inward to your belly and as you inhale consciously expand your abdominal muscles pressing in the floor beneath you. Feel your spine rising toward the ceiling. Then release the breath and feel your abdomen deflating and your spine dropping toward the earth once more. Take in the feeling of the letting go of the out-breath and the feeling of surrender to gravity. Become aware of the subtle power of gravity holding you to the earth.

In this place, feel your belly and recall a time when you were extremely hungry. Perhaps it is right now if it has been a while since you last ate. Perhaps it was a time when you were intentionally fasting. Perhaps it was a time when you were simply ravenous and yet you couldn't indulge your need to eat right away. Take time to recall the feeling of that strong hunger in your body and let your being become immersed in the feeling.

Then recall how you went about taking the steps to satisfy your hunger. Feel in your body the memory of the steps you took to acquire the food. What were your feelings as you went hunting about and selecting just the right food to satisfy your need? Recall the care and time you took in the preparation of the meal or the quality of the acceptance of the food that was served to you. Recall the very first bite and the feelings that it brought out in you as you began to feel the food go down inside you to meet the hungry feeling in your being. Recall the meal that followed that deep hunger, recall it completely from the first bite to the last.

Recall the variety of foods that were a part of the meal. Recall when in the meal you began to slow down and realize that you were very nearly satisfied. Remember the decision to keep eating until finally you knew it was time to stop. Were you saving room for dessert? Or did you have dessert anyway even though there was no room?

Now let yourself sink into the memory of your hunger being completely satisfied. For a moment, remember the feeling of being overstuffed. Take a deep breath and sigh, and let that go.

Come back into the current time and space and consider your hunger not just for food but for anything you might desire. What are those things in life you feel you must have in order to get through your life? Consider water, rest, touch, love, drugs, money, transportation, soaps, lotions, clothes, work, exercise, makeup, candy, ice cream, and toys. What are you constantly craving? How do you indulge it or resist it? Is it really necessary? Is it good for you? Do you have to have it? Does it nourish you?

What are you hungry for? Truly? Let yourself look at it. Do you need that? Could you do without? Honestly? What would that look like? Just for a moment, consider life without that thing that feeds you. What truly nourishes? Now let yourself have what you need, knowing that it is good, as it is good to be fed. It is right to be nourished.

Breathe deeply. Feel your belly press into the floor. Feel your spine rise to the sky. Fill up with breath deeper and deeper until you can't fill up any more, then hold it. Hold it. Hold it. Hold it. Hold on to it. Don't let it go. Don't let go. Hold on to it. Call to mind what you are hungry for and let the breath out, out, out, until you are completely empty and your spine has returned toward the floor.

Pause. Don't take a breath in, just wait. Wait. Don't do anything. Not even holding your breath now, just get out of the way and allow the air to come into your body all by itself. Watch it and feel the satisfaction that it brings as you fill up with nature. Then let it go again without effort. Breathe normally without control and just drift. Feel that all your needs have been met. Just float and drift on the waves of breath and life.

As you are ready, get up and share your experience with a friend. If there's no friend present, write it down, draw it, and remember it. Capture the insight that you gained through this experience with your own deep hunger.

Step Three: Your Personal Truth— Journey into Absolute Fire

On this third step of the journey we explore the realm of the Heart and Small Intestine. These are the meridians of absolute or sovereign Fire in the body, heartmind and spirit. This is where you take your throne and find the power to conduct the business of your realm.

Sit in a comfortable position and establish a connection with your breath. Gently close your eyes and focus inward on your body. See your in-breath going down into your inner body, and your out-breath coming out from your inner body. Feel the bottoms of your feet. Feel your sit bones pressing gently into the chair or floor.

Watch your breath for several cycles and then bring your attention to the area around your heart, behind the breastbone and to the left. See this area from the inside with your mind's eye. Allow yourself to simply be present with whatever bodily sensations you have in this area. There's no need to make anything up about what you feel or imagine anything in particular. Just simply open your awareness to what you do feel at this very moment.

Now send a wave of acceptance down and inward to your heart, fully appreciating it for all its long and steady service to your life. Appreciate its fundamental rhythmic beating that keeps your life flowing. Call to mind the very special nature of the heart muscle and its specialized intelligence.

It opens and closes rhythmically and precisely over and over again. It brings in venous blood (blood which has already circulated throughout your body) and sends it into the lungs for oxygenation, and brings in freshly oxygenated blood and sends it out as arterial blood back to circulate throughout your entire body.

The heart's intricate knowledge system brings in exact amounts of your precious life fluid and pumps it out again in equal volume. There are no central nervous system tissues in the heart. In other words, your brain does not control it; it does its job on its own.

In this place of awe and appreciation, take a moment to rest inward into Heart space. Breathe in, fill the area around the heart, and then let the breath go slowly and evenly (the heart muscle is attached to the diaphragm, so each breath actually moves the heart). Breathe this way slowly and deeply repeatedly quieting enough to be aware of the beating of your heart. And now consider your heart's truth—an idea, a feeling, a belief that you hold dear. Perhaps it has to do with your very identity as a person. Who are you? What is your heart's truth? What are you here on the planet to do? What is the truth you hold most dear?

As you ponder these questions, notice any voices that come into your head, voices of authority figures in your life, people who have influenced your outlook on life. Notice how their influence has shaped your own ideas. Recall how you accepted ideas from one source but not from another. Take a journey in your mind's eye to discover the shaping and the forming of your own unique sense of truth.

Recall a time when you held a truth that was in apparent opposition to the truth held by an authority figure in your life. How did you deal with this? Did you hide your truth to avoid conflict? As you recall this, notice the feelings in your heart. Did you question your own heart's truth and give way to the other person's point of view, allowing your own truth to be shifted? Did you hold your truth in and simply wait until that authority figure was no longer in your life? Did you confront the authority figure and let the chips fall where they may? At what point did you find the courage to stand in your own truth? And could you allow them to stand in their own opposing truth? Could there be more than one?

Breathe deeply and slowly and pay attention to the area around your heart. Notice the effects of this exploration on the quality of peace in your Heart. See yourself surrounded by people who share your truth, or are willing to allow you to have your truth even though it may be contrary to their position. Affirm your right to your own personal truth about who you are, what you believe, and what you hold dear. And affirm that same right to others as well. Appreciate your Heart, the central rhythmic intelligence of your life.

Take a few slow breaths and slowly come out of the meditation. Take time with your journal this time and write down or otherwise express your personal truth in some meaningful way. Then share that truth with a friend. After you have shared it with a friend, consider whom you might talk to who holds an opposing position. What would it be like to share your views with them? Take a few deep breaths at the thought, return your attention to your Heart, and just listen.

STEP FOUR: YOUR DEEPEST FEELINGS ABOUT LIFE AND DEATH— JOURNEY INTO WATER

At step four, we allow the elemental power of Water to come through us, as we drop into deep awareness of Bladder and Kidney functions. These powerful energies rest at the core of our being, governing the powerful action of the autonomic nervous system and all the deep instincts associate with life and death.

Take a comfortable position either lying on your back or sitting still. Calm your breath and look down and inward at your body. As you turn your consciousness inward, begin to direct your attention to the back of your body. Feel the back of your head, the back of your neck, all the way down your spine to your tailbone. Take time with this journey down your spine. Observe one vertebra at a time, and feel your back at each point. Remove judgment and open yourself to simply feel what presents itself at this time. As Tibetan Buddhism teaches us, be openly attentive to whatever arises. Apply this attentiveness to your awareness of your body.

After you focus on your spine, extend your awareness out to the sides of your back taking in the areas of the back of your shoulders, ribs, lower back, and buttocks. Apply the same attentiveness to these areas as you gave the spine. Breathe in and out slowly and deeply and notice the effects of the in-breath and out-breath on the sensations you feel in your body.

Move from the buttocks down into the back of your thighs, feeling the hamstrings, then the back of the knees and into the calves, and finally track the sensations of your body down into the bottom of your feet. Let your consciousness rest on the bottommost point of your foot, and imagine your in-breath coming in through this point. Feel the breath rising up your legs to the small of your back, and then release the out-breath down through the legs and out through this very same point.

Feel yourself deeply surrendered to the pull of gravity, and in this place move your attention toward your own birth into life. The story of your own birth that you heard from your parents, along with your own inner feelings about your arrival into life as a human being. Was it a happy day ... a challenging day ... a day of darkness? Were you welcomed into loving arms, a welcome addition to the human family? Or was your arrival met with fears and suspicions about whether your life was a good idea or not? Were you an unwanted, surprise child, or was your arrival planned? Consider this first moment and explore your feelings of being cherished and celebrated or barely tolerated. How does this moment show up in your own feelings about life?

Recall the memory of your face in the mirror. As you look at yourself, recall the face of your mother, your father. Let yourself sit and breathe with each image one at a time. Consider how your parents together brought you life. Do you see your mother's, your father's face when you look in the mirror at yourself? Remember their voices and the things that they said to you, and then recall your own voice, and the things you have said. Recall their mannerisms, the ones that please and the ones that annoy, and compare them to your own.

Take a deep breath. Imagine your parents as infants with your grandparents looking down at them. Do they smile? Are they stern? How do your parents feel about being alive? Is it a good thing to be alive? What is it to be alive? How does it feel to you? Do you have feelings about life that look the same as your parents' feelings?

Gently let the images of your parents drift away, and allow yourself to go further back, to grandmothers, and grandfathers, great-grandmothers, great-grandfathers ... to the stories, the family photo albums, recall your ancestry, your roots. See your genetic lineage as far back as you may, and take time to breathe in and out with your thoughts and feelings revolving around your ancestry and its history.

Let this go now and turn your attention to your children. If you do not yet have children, simply consider the idea of having children and all that that means to you. Consider what you will hand down to your children, the ways it will be an echo of what was handed down to you, and the ways in which it will differ.

Breathe in and breathe out, and consider life ... and death. What does it mean to you to have been given life? What does it mean to give life? And what of your own demise? Do you fear it? Do you court it? What does it mean to die ... to live? Consider your deepest innermost feelings about life and death.

Now, go inward and imagine your own passing. Will it be gentle? Violent? Do you cling to life, fighting death to the last breath? Or do you surrender to death gracefully and with ease? Is death a large and looming figure calling you into darkness, or a bright and shining light of life beyond life? What will your funeral be like? Can you see it? Will the ritual be grandiose, attended by many who mourn your passing... or will you pass away quietly without mention? Would you like to die alone on a hillside watching the sunset or the sunrise? Or will your death be sudden and unexpected?

Take time with these contemplations. Without judgment, simply notice your deepest innermost feelings about life and death. Tune in once more to your back body and gently recall your feelings at the start of the meditation. Notice any changes and reflect upon how your thoughts and feelings affect your body, your being.

Be gentle on yourself as you gradually pull yourself back into the current time and place. Slowly open your eyes and bring yourself to waking consciousness. Proceed to your journal and write or draw any impressions you have from this exercise. Keep them to yourself this time. You need not share these thoughts and feelings with anyone. At a later time, you may choose to, but for now, keep silence and let your inner strength grow through being dammed up. After journaling, practice a few vigorous exercises and feel yourself fully alive.

In the midst of your exercise, yell out "Hoka Hey!" It is a Lakota saying which means "it's a good day to die" which means it's a good day to live! Sit with that for a minute and consider what it means for you and your life... and death.

Step Five: Protection of All That Is Precious— Journey into Supplemental Fire

Supplemental Fire takes us through the realms of the Pericardium and Triple Warmer. These channels are said to the ministers to the throne in charge of regulations and communications.

Sitting comfortably once more take time to focus into your breath and become fully present. Allow yourself to be aware of the temperature of the room and your general level of comfort in your body. Notice the inflow and outflow of breath and see if you are aware of the rate of your heartbeat at rest.

Now imagine that you are on vacation staying in a small cabin in the mountains, surrounded by wilderness. You are there with a friend or two perhaps. Imagine the place fully and realize that you can relax here and there's no pressure on you to be anywhere but here or to do anything. There's a small fire stove and a simple kitchen you have stocked with all that you will need for the week. You have this time all to yourself to do with what you will.

The weather has been mild and gentle and you are feeling really good. One day you wake up and decide you want to go for a hike. Your friend isn't interested in joining you, so you decide to go ahead anyway by yourself. You pack a daypack, a lunch, and cheerfully set out on your hike. The weather is beautiful and sunny and mild and you set out with vigor and enthusiasm. Take a note to monitor the feelings in your body as you begin to experience the physical exertion. You easily climb up and over rocks and boulders in the trail and are gifted with spectacular views. Excited and exhilarated you walk a long, long way.

After a while, hunger pangs make themselves more and more obvious, and you decide to sit down and enjoy the lunch you packed. Satisfied with your meal you lean back and relax in the midday sun for a refreshing nap. When you wake you are still feeling good and you decide to continue to hike on a little ways further. You don't really have an idea what time it is, but it feels like there's lots of daylight left.

You hike on a few more miles, and almost without your noticing the weather begins to shift. There's a cloud or two that come into the sky. The sun is obscured and the air turns chilly. More clouds build up and as you stand on a high point and look around, you see the clouds really beginning to gather and darken. You decide you'd better turn back.

You didn't expect this turn in the weather, and you're a lot further away from the cabin than you thought. The weather worsens, getting colder and colder with winds from the north and heavier clouds. As you walk steadily along, you see snow beginning to fly.

Notice your breath and your bodily reactions to the cold. Note the steps you take to protect yourself from the weather and maintain your course. The storm is getting worse; the snow thickens from flurries into a blinding blizzard. It begins to accumulate on the ground. It's all you can do to make out the trail at your feet. You walk more hurriedly now, hoping to make it back to the cabin before nightfall.

The skies are dark from the storm, and the blowing snow obscures visibility. The accumulation gets deep, deeper than you could have imagined could ever fall in such a short time. The going gets tough now, but you plow steadily forward. Notice your body, how it is working in these conditions. You keep going, one foot in front of the other. Darkness falls, and you wildly consider whether you're going to ever make it back to the cabin. You are cold. Notice what part of your body most feels the cold.

Notice how you are dressed. Did you dress for the weather? Did you have an extra layer in your daypack to change into? How prepared were you for this change? Do you pat yourself on the back for being well prepared or are you angry with yourself for being ill prepared? For what it's worth, you consider your options. How will you survive this night?

Just as you begin to cast about for some way to protect yourself in the wilderness, you spy a glimmer of light up ahead. You move closer toward it. Beyond your wildest dreams you realize it is your cabin! Feel your heart rate when you first realize that you've made it. You go to the door and you reach for the handle and as you open the door you feel it pulled open and there is your friend ready to take you in. There's a crackling fire in the wood stove and you are welcomed back into the warmth and the light. You get out of your soaking wet clothes, your friend brings you a blanket and something hot to drink and eat. You snuggle up by the fire and recall the journey of your day, grateful to be safe and warm from the sudden storm. Breathe a sigh of relief and feel your body as it melts into the protection of warmth and friendship.

Take a few moments to come back to the room. Feel your body and mind in present time and space once more. Take a look at the question of how well you protect yourself. How well do you prepare for the un-expected? What warms your heart?

Take time to consider how it is you hold yourself dear, and how you take care of yourself in the face of the vicissitudes of life. What does it mean to protect yourself? How precious do you hold yourself to be?

STEP SIX: STANDING YOUR GROUND—A JOURNEY INTO WOOD

At this stage we take our stand with the energies of Gall Bladder and Liver, the hardworking first mate and the captain of the ship of your life. Gather up the energy you need to navigate the many passages of life.

This meditation is done in a standing position with the intention to strengthen your stance, sink your roots in the earth, and feel your branches reaching faithfully toward the sky. With this image in mind, stand with your feet shoulder width apart. Feel the bottoms of your feet. Feel grounded in the place where you stand. Feel your legs are slightly bent at the knee, giving you stability and flexibility. Make sure that your knees are not locked. Feel that your pelvis is free, with the tailbone slightly tucked under and forward. Feel your spine is loose and relaxed and held in a stable upright position. Your lower ribs are not protruding in the front, and your chest is slightly expanded. Your shoulders are dropped and your arms are resting gently at your sides. Your head is lifted up from the back at the nape of the neck, elongating your neck. Your chin is tucked slightly back. When we explore our qigong work in the next chapter, you will come to recognize this stance as the Wuji posture. This is a posture designed to stack your bones, give you a flexible upright posture, and connect you with the vastness and oneness of the entire universe.

Take several deep breaths and feel yourself rooted into the place where you stand. Notice a gentle swaying of your body as you breathe gently and deeply in and out. Feel suppleness in your body, all your muscles alive in a state of tonicity. Holding only the tension necessary to maintain your upright posture with ease—no more, no less.

Rest in this upright posture for several breaths, feeling the positive benefits of stillness and the confidence it brings you. As this feeling begins to permeate your being, allow your mind to become aware of the shape your body occupies in space, feeling the air around you. Feel your size and weight and contours and consider your strength.

Shift your weight to one foot and slowly slide the other foot out to widen your stance. Bend your knees more and tuck your tailbone forward between your legs. Feel as if you are riding on a horse. Allow your arms to rise up slightly to the side with your hands facing your hips. Develop an image of a Western gun fighter in your mind, and feel yourself getting ready to draw your guns.

In this posture, remember a time when someone crossed your path and deeply disturbed you. Feel the feelings of righteous anger that arose within you with this invasion of your territory. Recall whether you felt powerless at the time and the person walked all over you. Perhaps they were jealous of your territory and wanted a piece of it. Maybe they wanted what you had. Maybe their truth was in opposition to yours and they were working to dominate you with their point of view. Perhaps they wanted to intimidate you and threatened your very life. Perhaps they caught you unawares, coming in with honey and sugar and turning to vinegar, laughing as they stabbed you in the back.

Breathe deep. Allow yourself to feel the feelings in your body. Feel the bottoms of your feet. Feel your powerlessness as this person trespassed into your life. Now reimagine the situation and reclaim your power. Feel strength in your legs. Feel nimbleness and tonicity in your spine. Feel your arms in their power, ready to reach for your guns and defend your territory to the last. Notice the feelings that run up and down your body from the tip of your nose to the tip of your toes. Hold the person back. Hold your ground and do not allow them to walk all over you.

Breathe in, breathe out, and slowly resolve the situation. Stand firm in your place no longer threatened by the opposition. You have a right to your territory. You have a right to that which nourishes you. You have a right to your own sense of truth. You have a right to your own life, and your own death. You have a right to protect what is dear to you. And you have the strength to defend it. Feel your strength, and from your strength know your courage.

Come out of the meditation and take time to consciously write down or draw your experience of yourself, standing in your strength and holding your ground.

Reflections on the Journey

As you move through this elemental meditation sequence, see the progression from superficial to deep and back to the surface again, and see the importance of each facet in your life process. Where you find yourself deficient (a difficult condition to see) be gentle on yourself and simply seek out ways to acquire the necessary skills. Where you are excessive (a hard condition to admit) take the steps necessary to tone these aspects down. On the journey, cultivate an attitude of acceptance and change will come sooner. If you cultivate an attitude of intolerance toward what you may see as unseemly aspects of your being, you may find yourself fighting a losing battle with your greatest enemy—yourself. First accept yourself, and see why you behave the way you do. Only from this place can you make realistic and lasting positive change in your life.

Remember: what you resist persists. The harder you work to stave off what you most dread, the more likely it is to continue manifesting in your life. Make peace with this and all aspects of your being and you will see that as they soften they become weak, and as they become weak they can be overcome.

Elemental meditation, in the end, is a practice of liberation and freedom, freedom to feel what you feel and to find your own truth without fear of reprisal or the judgment of others. But this practice takes courage for you must be willing to look at yourself, listen to yourself, and discover ways of accessing yourself of which hitherto you were unaware. Other peoples' notions of right and wrong have been delivered so deeply into your psyche that the process of relearning them can be deeply challenging. In the end, you may find that you agree with what you have been taught. Rather than simply mimicing those who taught you, however, you will own the truth for yourself. When you come to this place, no one can get to you.

Breathe deeply. Take your time. Go at your own pace. And learn what that is. Learn to walk to the beat of your own drum. It's well worth the journey. Enjoy!

Chapter 10

Classical Movements and Qigong Practice

In this final chapter of our journey through the pathways of qi we make our way to our feet as promised to bring our study of qi meridian energy directly to our somatic, embodied experience. Rooted in the ancient wisdom and classical practices of qigong personal energy cultivation here you will find guidance on a full practice for total health and well-being.

Classical Qi Cultivation, Ancient Wisdom, Modern Applications

Qi is life force energy. *Gong* means to cultivate or to work. To practice qigong is to work with qi to cultivate the garden of life within. At the root of qigong practice are central teachings about the nature of the garden of life. The ancient Taoist sages were observers of the great vibrations of nature and the cosmos, and saw the practice of resonating with that vibration as the essence of health and balance.

We humans with our huge frontal cortex have mastered the art of objective thinking, separation, and putting things in neat little boxes. Qigong, the cultivation of life energy is ultimately the recognition of the oneness and interconnectedness of all things.

"The ultimate qigong goal is to connect directly into the force that runs the entire universe."[10] Tai chi and qigong masters know that the focused practice of these qi cultivating movements are central to self-healing. And the intention with which you practice directly relates to the benefits you will derive. Before you begin your practice of qigong it is important to ask the question, "Why do you want to learn qigong?" For you see, your intention is vital to your practice. Without a clear intention, there is no qigong.

The classical roots of qigong are deep in ancient history. It pre-dates tai chi, and itself is pre-dated by the deep mystical practices of neigong. It is a deep internal art. Walk into any modern martial art studio and watch the kicking and punching and blocking moves and you will immediately see the external martial arts in action.

The young and the new are always attracted to the external; the high and powerful kicks of Bruce Lee captivated the world. But the deeper initiation into the martial arts reveals that inside the external is the internal practice. And it is the internal practice that is most essential in the cultivation of life energy and the longevity, depth, and power of your life and practice.

A host of celebrated teachers profoundly influenced my practice and discovery of the secret and deep inner power of qigong cultivation. Deep at the root of qigong practice are a set of classical meditations, movements, and practices. These practices and the attitude and intention with which they are imbued are at the heart and soul of the health-giving

---

10   Roger Jahnke, *The Healing Promise of Qi* (New York: McGraw Hill, 2002), 12.

benefits of qigong. We will explore a range of classical movements and meditations and build a foundation for our practice. To deepen your ability to work with the pathways of qi, I will share with you my specialized qigong movement sequence, Meridian Gesture Qigong.

The Meridian Gesture Qigong Sequence

This sequence has been refined and crafted through my HeartMind Shiatsu training program over the last decade. It is rooted in the ancient understanding that the meridian location on the body directly correlates to the function of that meridian.

Meridian Gesture Qigong actualizes this understanding with a series of movements that articulate the meridian locations and acupoints, and stimulate qi energy flow, promoting balance and harmony throughout the meridian system.

The Meridians Gesture Qigong sequence specifically awakens, activates, and facilitates the smooth flow of qi through all the classical organ channels we have been studying. It works to clear blockages from acupoints along the way and to promote the health and balance of your internal systems rooted in your organ functions.

The body's organs are marvelously intelligent and skilled technicians each doing their assigned tasks without the need for conscious direction or oversight. The heart beats and pumps blood, the lungs bring in oxygen and release carbon dioxide, the stomach, spleen, pancreas, and intestines ingest and digest our food and nourishment, the liver performs more than four hundred complex chemical functions to maintain our energy and internal equilibrium, the kidneys purify the blood.

Each and every organ has its place and task and performs it tirelessly, day in day out. Our conscious mind is not needed to direct this action. But one thing our conscious mind can do that goes a long way is simply to appreciate these miraculous worker bees that conduct the business of our lives.

The organs love to be bathed in appreciation, gratitude, and love. When we direct our intentions in Meridian Gesture Qigong, we are honoring and acknowledging all these deep and working parts of our being. As a result, the whole system works better.

Do you recall a job in your early career where you received praise? How did that make you feel? If you're anything like me, it buoyed you up and made you want to do an even better job. The same is true for your internal organs. For all their complexity, they are also simple as children; a little positive recognition goes a long way.

The energy of life can be likened to a great river, continuously flowing from its headwaters to its delta at the sea. In the beginning it is gurgling and playful, jumping and bounding over boulders and rocks as it makes its way down from the mountains.

It leaps in thrilling white water chasms and waterfalls, it eddies in many a cataract and finds its way into lakes and over and under and around and through dams making its way to the broad plains where it becomes smooth and steady and flows inexorably to the sea.

Our qigong practice is much like this. We begin with warm-ups that are quite playful. As we leap over these first boulders of practice we begin to settle in, and eventually our movements slow into meditations and powerful flowing movements that flow from us internally like a great flowing river flowing unceasingly to the sea.

The energy builds up from start to end, and by the end of our practice we float upon the waves of the great ocean, deep, powerful, and connected to the great flow of life energy in the whole cosmos. As my favorite teacher Roger Jahnke once said, "Qi is the energy that keeps the earth circulating around the sun. The energy that can do that can heal your life!"

Basics of Qigong Practice

The following sequence of moving meditations form the basis of a full qigong practice. We start with warm-ups and classical qi awareness cultivation methods. We then move into Meridian Gesture Qigong. We complete with classical movements that consolidate and integrate the qi flow generated from the entire practice.

The components of a full practice that I will be leading your through are as follows:

1. Warm-ups

2. Classical qigong

3. Meridian Gesture Qigong

4. Completion and integration

1. Warm-Ups

The following warm-ups will bring you gently and fully into your practice. We will address Centrifuge, (Rapping on the Destiny Gate), Dropping the Post, Free Shaking, and Rolling Joints. You will be guided step-by-step through these warm up movements. As you practice, begin to become fully present and aware of your entire body.

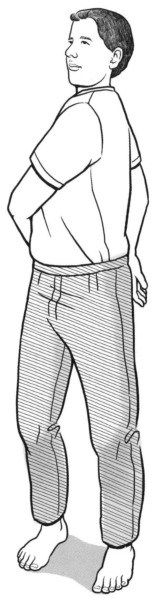

Figure 16: Rapping on the Destiny Gate.

CENTRIFUGE: "RAPPING ON THE DESTINY GATE"

- Start by standing upright with your feet slightly wider than your hips.

- Feel the vertical line of your body from the crown of your head to the root of your torso. Feel your weight evenly balanced on both feet.

- Begin to repeatedly turn your hips right and left.

- Allow your arms to be slack at your sides, and let them swing as a result of the twisting of your hips.

- Allow your arms to gently rap against your front and back body.

- Become aware of the specialized acupoint the "Destiny Gate" that is found on the midline of the spine between lumbar 2 and 3. The gentle rapping of your arms against your body as a result of the swinging of your hips opens your "Destiny Gate." This simple movement will have the action of freeing you up to be at your ease.

- Play with the rhythm, making the movements bigger, smaller, faster, slower. Notice how changes in speed can deepen your sense of relaxation and freedom in your body.

- As you are ready, wind it down, and come to stillness once more.

DROPPING THE POST: JIGGLING, WIGGLING, GIGGLING

- This is a joyous exercise that can really loosen up your whole body. Practice it with a sense of joy and childlike playfulness.

- Standing upright, first lift your heels and then drop back to floor with a jiggle.

- Repeat many times.

- Bend elbows, and with limp wrists jiggle your arms as you continue to drop the post.

- Release your jaw, open your mouth, and let out some noise.

- Alternate right and left feet, dropping the post in a jogging, jiggling motion.

- With open mouth, stick out your tongue. Keep jiggling and then let yourself giggle. Laugh out loud in playful abandon!

FREE SHAKING: PROGRESSIVELY SHAKE EVERY OUNCE OF FLESH IN YOUR BODY!

Dropping the post and jiggling and wiggling and giggling constitutes the classical set up for what we call "Free Shaking." In the following, I guide you through a "recommended sequence" so you can really begin to shake every part of your body. The sequence has no virtue in its own right, so I hope you eventually abandon it and really let your own shaking be free!

- Start by shaking hands, wrists, forearms, shoulders.

- Shake hips, legs, feet.

- Shake back, buttocks, thighs, calves.

- Shake cheeks, jowls, head, ears, eyes, nose.

- Shake ankles, feet, belly, chest.

- Let everything loose, and shake from your nose to your tailbone, like a wet dog.

Rolling Joints: Opening the Energy Gates

This classical sequence does ask you to settle down from the freedom of the shaking and follow a thorough step-by-step movement through every single working joint in your body. There are vital energy gates at every joint of the body. I like to think of these gates as the hinges. The meridian pathways can be likened to canals and the joints can be seen as elevation changes along the length of the canals. At each elevation change are a set of locks ships enter to be able to move from one section of the canal to the other. Keeping these energy gates open and in good working order is vital to the smooth flow of qi throughout the meridian channels. Perform these joint rolling exercises with the purpose of opening and lubricating the energy gates, releasing any blockages that may have accumulated due to tension, stress, and poor posture.

- **Simple head nods**—Start by nodding your head up and down, and feel this action all along the curve of the neck and down the spine. After going up and down several times, bring the head upright once more and then start dropping it from side to side, opening the sides of your neck.

- **Neck rotations**—From side to side head nods, bring your head upright, and then drop it forward and begin making "half circles" as you bring your chin up to one shoulder and then to the other. After several half circles, move into full circle making sure to go very gently to the back. Make three full circle in each direction and then bring your head upright once more.

- **Roll shoulders**—As your head rises out of the neck rotation sequence begin to roll your shoulders backward, then forward, together and then alternating right and left. Keep a smooth rotation going through the shoulders and notice any feelings of "gravel" in the shoulder joint. Move smoothly and gently to loosen this feeling of gravel in the shoulders. And as you do so, gently call to mind the many services that your shoulders do for your body, and with gratitude release any holding tension that may be present there.

- **Roll elbows**—Relax your shoulders, lift your elbows up and out to the sides, and begin to sweep your forearms in half circles, and then full circles. This will release the energy gates at your elbows.

- **Roll wrists, wiggle fingers**—Relax your elbows and then begin roll your wrists. Roll them back and forth and all around, changing direction many times. Then letting your wrists be still, gently wiggle your fingers.

- **Spiral Teacup**—One hand at a time, hold your palm up as if resting a tea cup there. Begin to spiral your hand around over your head and under your armpit keeping your palm upright so as not to spill a drop from your imaginary teacup. This action you will find involves your wrist, elbow, and shoulder in the spiraling action, and will even spiral down your torso to your hips. Let this action be fluid and smooth, and feel it through your entire body. Change directions a couple of times, and then repeat the spiral with the second hand. Adventurous folks may want to try spiraling teacups in both hands at the same time.

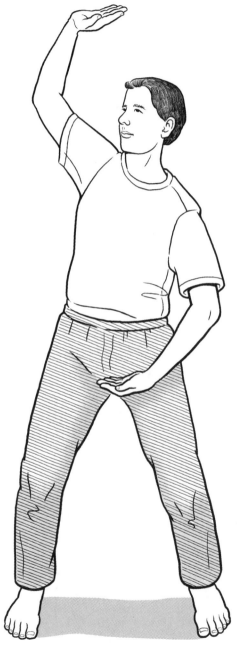

Figure 17A: Spiral Teacup.

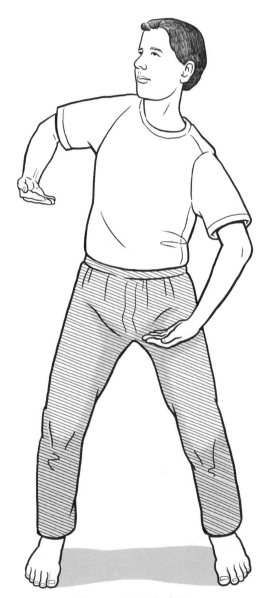

Figure 17B: Spiral Teacup.

- **Roll hips**—From spiral teacup you will find that you are moving your awareness down into your lower body. Now bring that awareness specifically to your hips, and with hands on your hips make wide swinging circles, first one direction and then the other. At some point, slow down the wide circling, and bring the movement into pelvic tilts, forward, back, right, and left, loosening your entire pelvic girdle and promoting the smooth flow of qi through these vital joints of the body that connect your legs to your torso.

- **Simple knee bends into knee circles**—Finish your pelvic tilts, and drop your hands down to your knees and begin simple, slow knee bends. After a few simply up and down movements begin to roll your two knees together in small circles, first one way and then the other.

- **One foot forward, plant big toe**—Roll ankle, knee, hip— after the knee bends, stand tall once more and bring one foot forward planting the ball mounts of the toes on the ground, beginning to roll the hip, knee, and ankle, rotating down through each and every toe. Make circles one way and then the other, changing directions many times.

- **Lift one foot, balance**—Rotate ankle, spread toes—If you are not certain of your ability to balance on one foot, move behind a chair and steady yourself as you lift one foot and make circles with the ankle. To get this action right, imagine that you are "drawing a circle" with your big toe, as if a felt-tip marker were on the tip of your big toe. Draw a nice smooth circle and reverse the direction several times.

2. Classical Qigong Practice

After being sufficiently warmed up, we now take our qigong deeper into our being with a series of classical practices. Honoring the Three Treasures, Radiant Heart Gesture, Seven Directions, Meditation, Plies, Wuji (in posture, breath, and mind), Small Heavenly Circle Meditation, and Stance Training all have their place in our practice, and each yield rich, extraordinary gifts in activating the qi essence throughout body, heart-mind, and spirit.

HONORING THE THREE TREASURES

The Three Treasures constitute the foundation understanding that is at the core of all effective qigong practice. And though this comes from China, and classical Taoist observations of nature and the universe, it really speaks to a universal truth, founded on a very deep common sense. The Three Treasures are called by the distinct names jing, qi, and shen, and they are all considered to be various aspects of the manifestation of life energy.

Jing is the most dense expression of life energy, and the source energy from which all springs forth. It is physical in nature and can be observed, touched, held, and manipulated directly through physical intervention. It can be considered as manifesting in our very DNA, the genetic material that has made you who you are in this lifetime in this body. The sperm and the egg are considered direct manifestations of jing, and this jing essence is the essential building block of our physical being. Closely related to jing are the fundamental substances of blood and bodily fluids. These fluid components of human life are vital to daily functioning.

Qi is more energetic in nature than jing. It is less physical though the physical is imbued with qi and we can read the quality of qi through our five senses. In a simple and direct way, qi can be compared to air. It is the medium of the atmosphere in which all life on earth thrives.

It's notable that despite its presence, it is not something you can generally see with the naked eye. It is also found in liquid medium of water and the solid medium of rock and soil. The Chinese proverb puts it into perspective: "Fish cannot see water, humans cannot see qi." From this you can conceive that qi is the medium in which we humans "swim."

The third treasure is shen. Shen is the most ethereal of the three, equated with spirit, it extends through the vast reaches of space and may be discerned as light, the life giving energy that emanates from the stars and reflects off all the heavenly bodies. In human expression, we see shen in the expression of emotions, thoughts, and higher levels of consciousness.

To awaken an awareness of the Three Treasures in a very simple way, try the following movements while opening your consciousness to the three levels of being.

- **Jing**—Earth, the ground beneath us. Stamp your feet, feel all that is beneath you. Gently tap your body and feel the flesh of your being. Look in the mirror and see your size, shape, gender and ethnicity, the inheritance you were born with. Feel the tissues of your body, the fluids of your body, the circulation and rhythm of blood flowing through your body.

- **Qi**—The fields of life, the air that surrounds us. Twist right left, up down, back, front, and feel all that surrounds you in these fields of life. Qi exists here in the middle realm between heaven and earth, between spirit and matter. Take big, deep breaths in and out and feel the edge where air becomes a part of you on the inhale, and that which was inside you leaves you on the exhale and becomes a part of the air that surrounds you.

- **Shen**—Heaven, the vast reaches of space and the light of the heavenly bodies. Sweep your arms overhead and feel all that is above you. Open your perception of the vast reaches of space and the mystical quality of all that is unseen and lies beyond common five sensory awareness.

RADIANT HEART GESTURE: DANCING HEAVEN TO EARTH

The Radiant Heart Gesture opens the whole body, and helps you begin to deepen into the qigong state of consciousness. This is a relaxed but alert state of being in which awareness is heightened and qi can flow optimally. Qi flows best when any unnecessary tension is removed from the body. The goal here is to do all moves with a minimum of effort. In fact, cultivating a kind of "floating feeling" is ideal. And in the end you begin to experience a kind of "non-doing" or weightlessness. With advanced experience of the work, you can arrive in a space where you seem to be observing the movements without apparently exerting any effort to do them at all. It's as if the movements are being done through you. The famous football quarterback Joe Namath was once quoted as saying, "I don't play football. Football plays itself through me." This statement gets close to describing what the qigong state may feel like for you.

- In the Radiant Heart Gesture we cultivate our awareness of yin and yang, through a felt sense of the body's magnetic field. Below I will describe two ways of performing the Radiant Heart Gesture, one activating the yang flow and the other the yin flow. At first cultivating an awareness of the magnetic field may require a bit of good old fashioned imagination, but over time you may find that you feel a palpable quality of energy you might characterize as magnetic. To call this into your imagination, first realize that the magnetic field is real, and it does surround your body, emanating most strongly from the area of your heart.

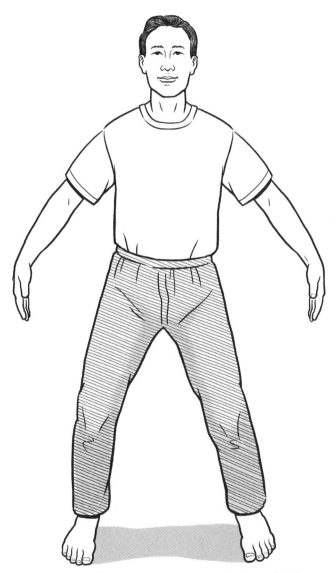

Figure 18: Radiant Heart Gesture: Gathering of Light—
Pulling Down the Heavens 1.

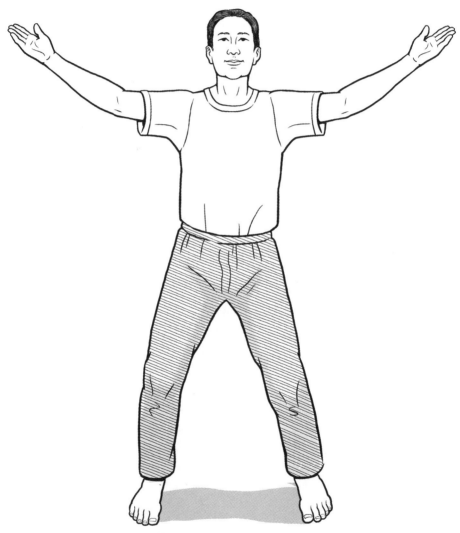

Figure 19: Radiant Heart Gesture: Gathering of Light—
Pulling Down the Heavens 2.

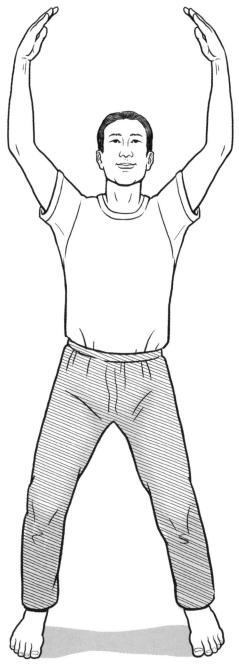

Figure 20: Radiant Heart Gesture: Fountain of Life 1.

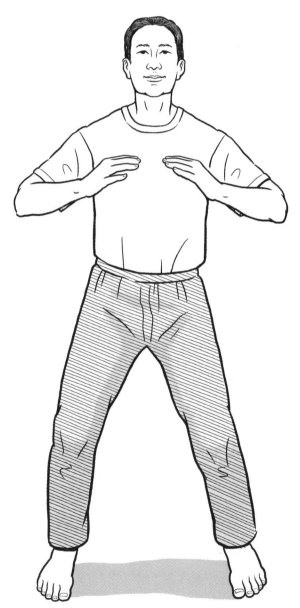

Figure 21: Radiant Heart Gesture: Fountain of Life 2.

- Recall too that magnets are made up of the oscillation of energy between the positive and negative magnetic poles. These positive and negative energies are correlated to the jing and the shen we discussed above, or more simply as yin and yang. Yin, the negative pole, is related to the earth below us and yang, the positive pole, is related to the heavens above us.

- Finally, the shape of a magnetic field is called a torus, which for the purposes of this exercise may be visualized to be much like the shape of a round piece of fruit. First, standing in an easy upright posture, call to mind the shape of an apple or orange, and activate your awareness of this shape as a large, luminous sphere of light or magnetism, emanating from your center and surrounding your entire body.

- **Yang: Gathering of Light**—Pulling Down the Heavens— yang energy is of the heavens, and moves down through the core of the body, dispersing down into the earth. As you breathe in, sweep arms down toward the earth and out to your sides, gathering in soil, water, wind. Then continue to sweep your arms up toward the heavens and imagine that you are gathering in the light of the sun, moon, and stars. As your arms reach high above you, slowly begin to lower them down along the midline of your body as you gently breathe out.

- **Yin: Fountain of Life**—Yin energy of the earth moves up through the core of your body, shoots up into the sky over your head, much like a geyser or fountain, and then disperses into the sky above and sprinkles back to the earth. Breathing in, draw your hands together up along the midline of the body and up overhead into the sky above, shooting up like a strong fountain of water. As your hands reach your full height, breathe out, sweep your hands out to the sides, and back down to the earth, wiggling the fingers like water droplets from the fountain dispersing in the sky on its way back to earth.

- Practice alternating Fountain of Life and Pulling Down the Heavens as you twist your body right and left, sweeping arms through the entire torodial magnetic field of the body, heartmind, and spirit. Let your knees bend and straighten as you sweep your arms, creating sinking and rising movements to enhance the overall flow of qi through the luminous magnetic field of the body.

SEVEN DIRECTIONS MEDITATION

The Seven Directions Meditation is a time honored practice to assist you in discovering your centerpoint. A Taoist proverb reads "At the center of every turning wheel is a point that does not move." Finding this still point is at the core of remaining balanced in a world that is often "spinning" at a rapid pace. Please go through this practice slowly and take time at each station to open the windows of your perception to whatever may show up for you.

- Sit quietly. Tune into your breath. Close your eyes.

- With your mind's eye, see all that is beneath you. Take note. Breathe in, breathe out.

- Turn your gaze, see all that is below you. Take note. Breathe in, breathe out.

- Turn your gaze to the right, see all that is to your right. Take note. Breathe in, breathe out.

- Turn your gaze to the left, see all that is to your left. Take note. Breathe in, breathe out.

- Turn your gaze to the back of you, see all that is behind you. Take note. Breathe in, breathe out.

- Turn your gaze toward the front of you, see all that lies ahead. Take note. Breathe in, breathe out.

- Breathe in, breathe out. Take note. Below, above, right, left, back, front ...

- Turn your gaze inward. See what is in your center. Take note. Breathe in, Breathe out.

PLIES

These exercises actually derive from the ballet. Though they are not strictly taught in classical qigong methods, I have found them to be extremely effective in developing consciousness of the body in motion. They serve the purpose of enhancing personal awareness of your centerpoint while in movement, and for establishing a deep felt sense of alignment in the bones and joints and coordination of the muscles of the hips, knees, ankles, and feet.

Standing upright, squeeze the muscles of the buttocks to create a lateral rotation of the femur in the hip socket. This is known as a "turn out" in ballet. You may recall seeing ballerinas walking with their feet turned out, instep facing forward. But what is important to note here is that the turn out needs to start in your hips and the feet must not be turned out further than the hips. The goal is to laterally rotate the femur and then bring the knees, ankles, and feet in alignment with that rotation, not further.

The plie is then performed by bending the knees to lower your center of gravity, while keeping the torso upright. Take care to bend the knees out directly over the big toes or even middle toes. This alignment is critical and will help you maintain proper alignment, tone, and integrity of the lower body, an essential component in the art of balance.

There is an entire series of standing ballet exercises that can be used in enhancing your qigong standing practice. For its part, the plie is the core method with which you need to become familiar. As you continue through the standing exercises below, continue to pay close attention to the alignment of hips, knees, and ankles in all your movements and postures.

WUJI: THE MOTHER POSTURE OF QIGONG

You'll recall that in our study of yin and yang we quoted the proverb: "One, the universe divided, becomes two, yin and yang, opposites that make the whole." Well, *wuji* is the "one" in this quote; the "whole." Yin and yang are the two parts of the *tai chi*, the "great chi" often translated as the "great ultimate." Yin and yang are contained within wuji. And at the same time, wuji represents the full undifferentiated wholeness before the division into yin and yang.

And so, wuji is the primordial, undifferentiated, ever-present energy of the universe. It is the source and the essence of all things manifest and potential. It is oneness. It is non-dual. Practicing the posture, we practice melting/dissolving into the non-dual.

It is a standing meditation, that is profound in its application, scope, and impact. In traditional qigong training, it is my understanding that this is the only exercise practiced in the entire first year of training. Imagine not learning any other exercises to practice for one whole year but standing still!

In your standing still, you will note three areas of focus: your posture, your breath, and your mind. Start with posture, then bring in the focus on your breath, and finally watch your mind. Take your time. There is nowhere to go, nothing to do, nothing to achieve, nothing to prove, no one to please. Simply drop in, and breath by breath, move yourself deeper into stillness.

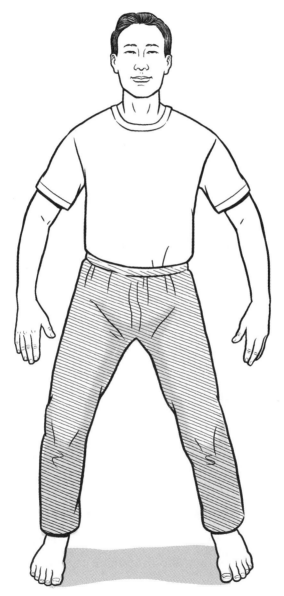

Figure 22: Wuji.

Wuji—Postural Awareness

- Stand with your feet just wider than your hips.

- Parallel your feet, as if you are wearing cross-country skis, with the skis in parallel tracks.

- Gently bend your knees, aiming them directly out over the middle toes.

- Feel your tailbone sink toward the earth. If a line were dropped down from your tailbone it would touch a spot exactly in the center between your two feet.

- Feel "marionette strings" attached to your elbows pulling them up and out to the sides. Hands will face obliquely toward the back.

- Feel your spine rising up to the heavens. The back of your head lifts, your chin tucks in slightly.

- There is a gentle lifting in your sternum. Your belly is relaxed and open.

- Allow the tip of your tongue to rest on your top palate behind the top teeth. Eyes are just barely open or gently closed. Focus inward.

Wuji—Breath Awareness

- Standing in the posture of wuji, turn your attention to your breath.

- Follow the breath down into your inner body.

- Imagine that your body is like a balloon. The inhalation enters, fills the center, and from there expands out in all directions. The exhalation relaxes, and the balloon shrinks back to the center.

- Slow the breath down to "turtle's breath"—four cycles per minute.

- Practice "six-sided breathing." From the center, expand the torso front and back, right and left, top and bottom. Creating space for all the internal organs. Recall your practice in the Seven Directions meditation to enhance your experience of this breathing awareness.

Wuji—Mind Focus

Let the mind be as the sky and the thoughts and feelings as the clouds. Just as the sky does not cling on to the clouds, your mind need not cling on to your thoughts and feelings. Allow the thoughts and feelings to float through your mind, like clouds through the sky. Sometimes the sky is full of clouds, sometimes it is clear and blue. Be not concerned, let the thoughts and feelings be and follow none of them, just let them come and go.

SMALL HEAVENLY CIRCLE MEDITATION

The Small Heavenly Circle meditation is also known as Microcosmic Orbit. It is an ancient Taoist meditation that has been handed down for generations. It is particularly focused on opening the two central vessels of the body. These vessels are two of the eight extraordinary vessels and are the only extraodinary vessels that have acupoints of their own. The remaining six vessels all use points along the regular channels, interconnecting the system from superficial to deep. These two central vessels begin at the perineum, the midpoint between the genitals and the anus at the bottom of the torso. One vessel runs up along the midline of the front body and ends at the lower lips. We call this the Sea of Yin. The other runs up along the midline of the back body, over the crown of the head and down the forehead through the nose to end at the upper lip. We call this the Sea of Yang.

Much like meridians, these vessels run right through the centerline of the body and have acupoints of their own. Of note though, these are not considered to be regular channels. As we discussed earlier, these vessels connect us deep into the constitutional layers of health, and can be used to great effect to tap into the very origins of life itself. A helpful analogy to draw between meridians and vessels is to think of rivers and reservoirs. The meridians are like rivers, and the vessels are like reservoirs. In times of flood, we fill the reservoirs so that we might have a resource to draw upon in times of drought.

Your extraordinary vessels are the reservoirs of your constitutional qi, your original endowment of life energy. As such they are the place you can go to to draw strength in times of difficulty, and to connect to the reason and purpose for your life. The Small Heavenly Circle meditation gives you access to the source qi as it manifests in these two "extraordinary" midline vessels, and as such can be seen as a primary tool in the work of self-healing.

One more note to take to heart, the front vessel is known as the conception vessel and we recognize it as the Sea of Yin. All the yin energies of the body can be connected into this vessel. And the back vessel is known as the governor vessel, the Sea of Yang. Here all the yang energies of the body can be accessed and addressed. And so, the Small Heavenly Circle meditation serves to balance yin and yang in the body and in your life. Follow along these vessels and their major points as you open the awareness of qi energy flowing through the seas of yin and yang, promoting inner balance and and deep harmony within you.

- See a bright pearl of light at the third eye yin tang point between your eyebrows. Build the energy and light there.

- Draw the pearl of light down the bridge of your nose, into the tip of your tongue, down your throat and into your heart center. Let the energy and light build there.

- Draw the pearl down from your heart center along the midline of the front body, past the navel into the lower abdomen, the lower *t'an t'ien*, your "energy ocean" or "elixir field." Let the energy and light build there.

- Continue to stream the energy down the front midline from the third eye to the t'an t'ien.

- From t'an t'ien, draw the pearl of light down to the root chakra at the perineum, midway between the genitals and the anus.

- From the root, draw the pearl of light back to the tailbone.

- From the tailbone, draw it up the midline of the back body, to the *ming men*, "destiny gate," Governor Vessel 4, between the lumbar vertebrae 2 and 3.

- Continue to draw it up the spine to the back heart, to the base of the neck, base of the skull, and then up to *bai wei*, "meeting point of one hundred meridians," GV 20, at the crown of the head.

- Feel the energy bright and strong at bai wei and draw it forward to connect once more with yin tang, the third eye.

- Having completed one full circle, now continue, circulating the energy down through the midline of the front body, and up the midline of the back body. Repeat over and over.

STANCE TRAINING: BUILDING STABILITY, STRENGTH, ENDURANCE, AND COURAGE

Stance training takes what you have learned from plies and the wuji posture and amplifies this practice into a full body discipline that will yield incredible benefits for you in the areas of strength, stability, balance, endurance, and courage.

This exercise sequence can be quite intense; you should allow yourself a chance to gradually work up to its full expression. At the same time, monitor your own level of readiness for this practice. At first you may only hold each posture for one or two breath cycles. Gradually you can lengthen the amount of time you spend in each position, up to eight minutes for each.

Depending on your available time for practice, you will need to watch the clock and determine how this sequence fits into your overall practice. It can be used interchangeably with the Meridian Gesture Qigong sequence. Yet it also complements that sequence. You will see a great deal of overlap and redundancy between these sequences. This repetition is intentional and purposeful and will ultimately deepen your practice overall.

- **Horse Stance—base posture:** This is basically wuji posture but a little wider and with the image of riding horseback.

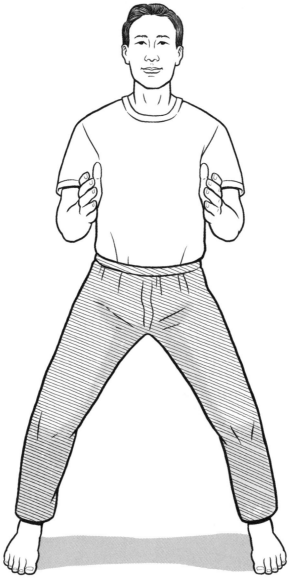

Figure 23: Horse Stance.

- **Forward Stance—right and left:** A classic 60/40 stance, hips squared to front foot. Front leg bent, back leg straight. Come back to horse, repeat to other side.

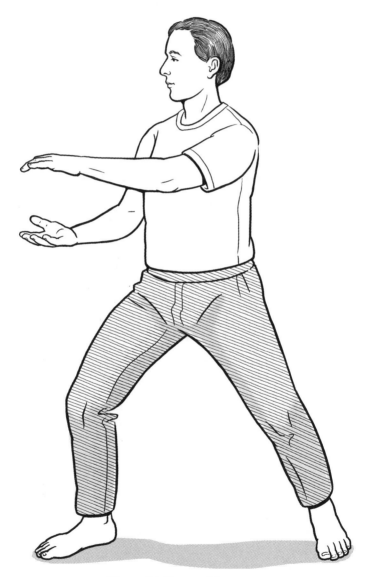

Figure 24: Forward Stance.

- **Toe Stance—right and left:** All weight on one foot, hips turned 45 degrees toward unweighted leg. Toe of unweighted leg touches the ground with knee bent. Come back to horse, repeat to other side.

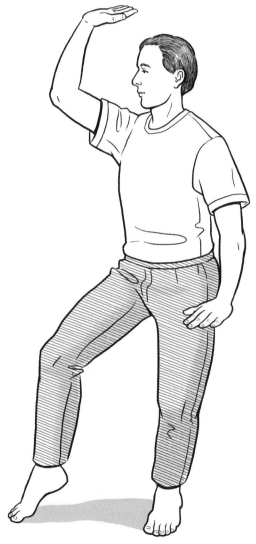

Figure 25: Toe Stance.

- **Heel Stance—right and left:** All weight on one foot, hips turned 45 degrees toward unweighted leg. Heel of unweighted leg touches the ground, this leg is completely straight. Come back to horse, repeat to other side.

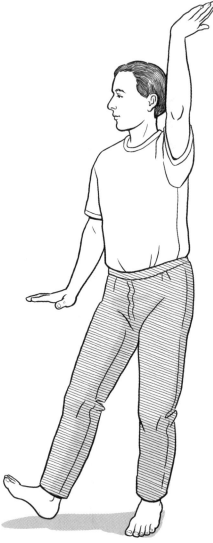

Figure 26: Heel Stance.

- **Cross Stance—right and left:** All weight shifts to one foot. The other foot sweeps behind, crossing over the midline. Ball mount of rear foot accepts half the weight. Bending knees, the rear knee aims toward front foot. Come back to horse, repeat to other side.

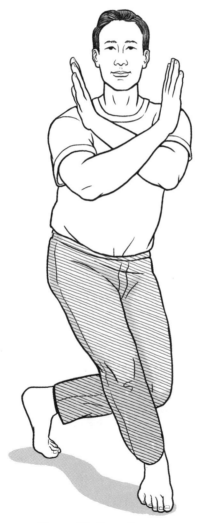

Figure 27: Cross Stance.

- **Deep Stance—right and left:** Place all weight on one foot while bending knee and dropping center of gravity low. The other foot slides out away from the midline as far as possible, into this deep stance. Arms swing out over extended leg. Switch sides with a "ki-ai!" yell, straightening the bent leg, and bending deep to the other leg, swinging the arms in a full arc and out over the extended leg on the other side. Repeat several times. End in Deep Horse.

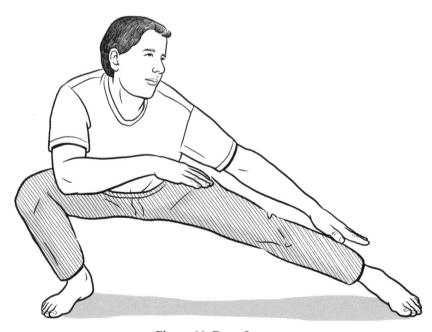

Figure 28: Deep Stance.

- **Standing White Crane—right and left:** Standing on one leg, the arms lift up wide over the head, as the knee of the un-weighted leg rises, toes pointed toward knee of standing leg. Gaze straight ahead. Lower arms and leg together. Then raise arms and lift the second leg. Repeat going from side to side in rhythmic fashion.

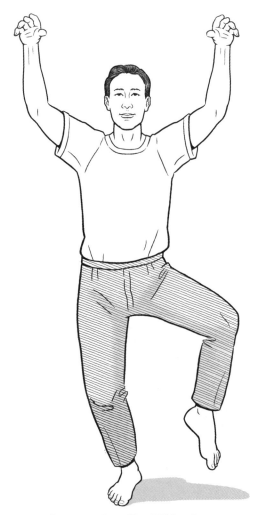

Figure 29: Standing White Crane.

- **Bear Stance—right to left:** Feet comfortably parted, just wider than hips, turn them inward or pigeon-toed. Sink your weight onto one knee, bending that knee and turning your hips 45 degrees toward the unweighted leg. Come up smoothly and shift to other side. Hold hands like bear paws in front of the chest at shoulder height.

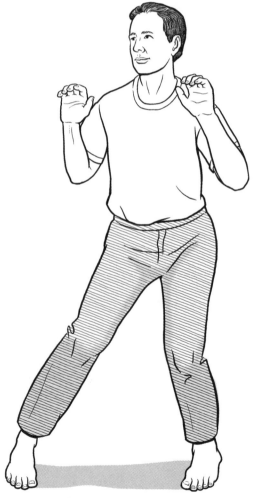

Figure 30: Bear Stance.

3. Meridian Gesture Qigong

Before I guide you through the Meridian Gesture Qigong sequence, it is good to recall once more the sequence of the one meridian flow, and review each of the meridian starting and ending points. Fresh from this review, we will get right into the qigong gesture for each meridian.

CIRCADIAN RHYTHM: MERIDIANS AND THE 24-HOUR CLOCK

- Lung, 3–5 am; Large Intestine 5–7 am;

- Stomach 7–9 am; Spleen, 9–11 am;

- Heart, 11 am–1 pm; Small Intestine, 1–3 pm;

- Bladder 3–5 pm; Kidney, 5–7 pm;

- Pericardium, 7–9 pm; Triple Warmer, 9–11 pm;

- Gall Bladder, 11 pm–1 am; Liver, 1–3 am.

CLASSICAL TRAJECTORY OVERVIEW

Where one channel ends, the next begins nearby, creating one continuous flow:

- Lung begins just lateral to the second rib and ends in the thumb.

- Large Intestine begins in the index finger and ends at the nose.

- Stomach begins at the eyes and ends at the second toe.

- Spleen begins in the big toe and ends in the side ribs under the axila.

- Heart begins in the axila and ends in the pinky finger.

- Small Intestine begins in the pinky finger and ends at the ear.

- Bladder begins at the eyes and ends at the pinky toe.

- Kidney begins in the bottom of the foot and ends at the clavicle.

- Pericardium begins outside the breast and ends in the middle finger.

- Triple Warmer begins on the ring finger and ends at the eyebrow.

- Gall Bladder begins at the outer eye and ends at the fourth toe.

- Liver begins on the great toe and ends in the ribs just under the breast.

- Lung begins on the chest just lateral to the second rib ...

MERIDIAN GESTURE QIGONG

The HeartMind Meridian Gesture Qigong sequence follows the daily cycle of energy flow beginning with Lung and working through each meridian in sequence to Liver. This sequence affirms the flow of the one meridian and its many points and facets in the twelve organ networks of the body. It is firmly rooted in the classical understanding that once you know the function the organ network performs you can nearly predict where the meridian line will be on the surface of the body. And as you accentuate that line on the surface of the body you are activating and supporting the smooth flow of qi in that meridian system to maintain and sustain its optimal functioning. The gestures of the meridian channel aspects that follow are the foundation movements and mindset of the Heartmind Meridian Twelve Qigong sequence, especially developed to open and stimulate the life energy in the one meridian and its twelve channels to increase consciousness, healthy balance, and flow.

THE LUNG CHANNEL GESTURE

As you strike a pose that stretches all the points along the Lung channel from the pectoralis muscle to the thumb, you will see that this pose deeply and directly relates to the movement of breath in and out of your body.

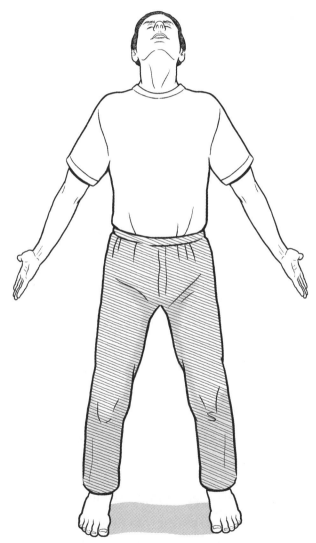

Figure 31: Lung Channel Gesture.

- Start in the wuji posture. As you exhale, slowly fold forward, bending your knees, shifting your belly back in space, dropping your head, and bringing your hands forward almost touching thumbs together at the midline.

- Breathing in, slowly rise up with thumbs leading the hands and arms out to the side and behind you. Open your chest skyward and stretch your thumbs to the back. This position stretches the entire Lung meridian, and as you perform it you will find that you automatically take in a large breath filling your lungs with air.

- After stretching fully open, slowly reverse the action, exhale, close down your chest once more, drop your head, and nearly touch your thumbs together in front of you.

- On the next inhale, open once more, and on the exhale, close to the front.

- Repeat the entire exercise several times.

- On the inhale; breathe in white, the pure qi of the universe.

- On the exhale breath out all your gray, murky qi that you no longer need. Breathe out your sorrow and loss. Give it back to the universe.

- Let this gesture build your awareness of the breath, the most basic fundamental rhythm of the body, heartmind, and spirit. Shower your lungs with gratitude and unconditional love.

The Large Intestine Channel Gesture

When you strike a pose that stretches out the entire flow of this channel, you find yourself pointing down to the ground with the index finger while at the same time lifting your nose up to the sky. This is a posture you might assume if you were pointing down at a malodorous pile of matter that had clearly just emerged from some animal's large intestine. This follows right after the Lung gesture, in the Meridian Gesture Qigong sequence.

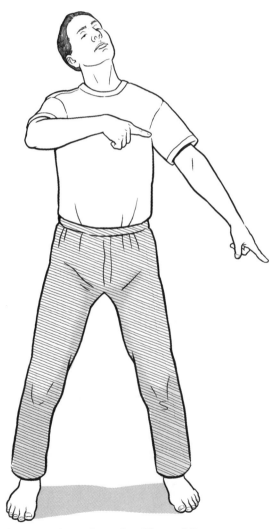

Figure 32: Large Intestine Channel Gesture.

- As you stand tall on the last exhale of the Lung gesture, make light fists and point both index fingers down toward the ground.

- Slowly shift your hands to point down to the left. The left index finger particularly points strongly down to the ground, as if pointing at a dung pile.

- The right index finger then points toward the left index finger, and draws a line up along the Large Intestine meridian line from the index finger to the nose and beyond.

- Point the right index finger strongly toward the heavens, while the left index finger continues to point to the earth. Repeat the affirmation: "I graciously let go of that which no longer serves me."

- Sweep the right hand now down toward a dung pile on the earth off to your right, and let the left index finger sweep over and draw the line up along the Large Intestine meridian line on the right arm, from the index finger to the nose and beyond.

- Sweep it up and out toward the heavens, and point it down again at the left side.

- Repeat this sweeping gesture many times to each side. Affirm the Large Intestine in its task of letting go of all that you no longer need.

- Return to wuji posture and feel the benefits of the movements.

THE STOMACH CHANNEL GESTURE

As you strike a pose that activates this entire channel, you will find that you are much like a picture of a hunter-gatherer warily stalking your prey. The classic Meridian Twelve Qigong movement is drawn from the yoga posture of Warrior 1 and speaks to the strong energy that governs the essential function of appetite in our human life.

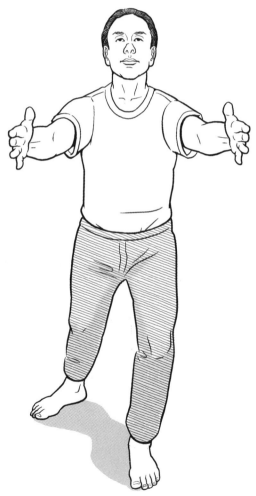

Figure 33: Stomach Channel Gesture.

- From wuji, shift your weight smoothly onto the right foot and lunge forward with the left foot.

- Turn your right foot to 45 degrees keeping the right leg straight.

- Square the hips forward toward the left, with left knee bent. Bend forward at the hips, bringing the hands down along the left leg to the left foot.

- Sweep your hands out in front of you, and stretch out through your arms as you slowly raise your torso to an upright position, with your arms projecting overhead in line with your ears. Your left leg remains bent, right leg straight forming a strong foundation for what is known in yoga as the Warrior 1 posture.

- As if holding something between your palms, bring them down to trace the Stomach channel from face to throat, to chest, to belly, and then forward bend down the leg to the foot, and sweep out to the ground in front of you once more.

- As you raise your arms this time, imagine that you are growing a tree from the roots up the trunk to the branches to the fruit. Then you are harvesting that ripe fruit and bringing it down to nourish your whole being, head, heart, and hara (center).

- Sweep down the leg a third time, and repeat the entire gesture.

- After stretching tall, bring the energy between your palms down to the heart level and switch your feet. Repeat the gesture three times on the second side.

With each of the sweeping gestures, imagine pulling that which you want and need down through the Stomach meridian channel. Note how the channel flows through the head, the heart, and the belly. It is nice to think of these as the three stomachs, for indeed we have appetite in all three areas: intellectual, emotional, and physical. And all appetite is the domain of Stomach channel. Enjoy this gesture with all the gusto you can muster.

THE SPLEEN/PANCREAS CHANNEL GESTURE

Spleen/Pancreas is all about nourishment, sweetness, and goodness. If you strike a posture that articulates this entire channel you will find that your body takes on an aspect that is provocative and inviting, holding the promise of sweet nourishment. To practice the movement that supports Spleen function, do the following:

- From wuji, step your feet slightly wider and turn out your hips, knees, and feet about 45 degrees.

- Sweep your arms up and out to the sides and down toward the ground.

- As you sweep toward the ground, plie at the knees, and bring your left hand to the earth as if to pick a ripe strawberry.

- Rise up, bring the "strawberry" to your mouth while shifting your weight onto the right foot, and bringing your left foot forward, presenting the Spleen channel from the big toe up to the breast.

- With your left hand at your mouth, enjoying the strawberry, let your right hand rub your belly in a clockwise direction.

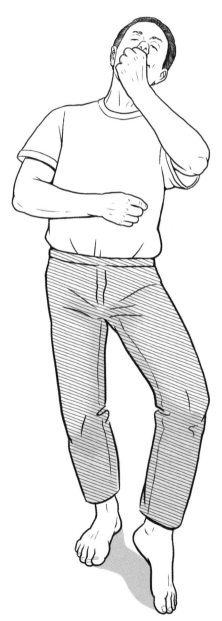

Figure 34: Spleen/Pancreas Channel Gesture.

- After a moment, sweep the hands up, out, and down once more. Return the feet to a plie to descend easily to pick another strawberry.

- This time, use your right hand to bring the strawberry to your mouth. Let the left foot take your weight and bring the right foot forward to present again to the Spleen.

- Enjoy flowing from right to left repeatedly each time deepening the sweet feeling. Let yourself connect to a "happy for no reason" feeling, and be aware that balance is required for this movement just like it is in the regulation of the rise and fall of blood sugar.

The Heart Channel Gesture

This gesture should be performed in slow and flowing movements to fully activate the heart channel. As you practice, you may recall the posture of those praising God or the spirit world with the uplifting feelings of love and joy.

- From wuji, allow the backs of your hands to float toward one another, in front of your hara.

- Slowly draw them up the midline of your body, passing the heart center, the throat, the third eye, and rising above your head.

- Slowly open them out to the sides, palm up, while gazing heavenward with a slight backward tilt of your head, holding a golden ball of qi overhead.

- Begin to turn right and left, twirling the qi ball above your crown.

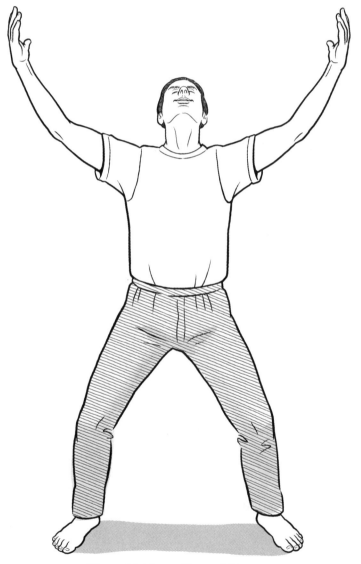

Figure 35: Heart Channel Gesture.

- After a time of twisting right and left, turn to face front and raise your palms directly over your head as if they were showerheads showering a deep red light down onto your crown.

- Bring your gaze to horizontal, bend at the knees, sink down toward the earth, and feel that deep red light flowing from your crown down to your feet.

- After several breaths, gradually turn your palms toward the heavens once more, leading with the pinky fingers, like a lotus flower blossoming under the sun. Expand your chest and arms feeling that you are connecting with the vastness of the entire universe.

- After several breaths, slowly sweep your hands down toward your sides and pause, feeling the energy of the Heart channel activated and coursing through your being.

- Let the pause be dynamic as you flow continuously into the Small Intestine gesture.

THE SMALL INTESTINE CHANNEL GESTURE

Taking a look at the entire meridian from the first to the last point, we make the gesture of knifing the hand and arms down through space until bringing them alongside the body, turning the head to look back over one shoulder. When seen from behind, this gesture will expose the entire surface of the meridian channel. And the mental focus of the gesture should carry the quality of communicating the statement, "Get back!" or to quote scripture, "Get thee behind me!" The Small Intestine must separate the pure from the impure, and this gesture shows how the surface trajectory of the meridian and the actions of the muscles through which it runs serves to support and illustrate that function.

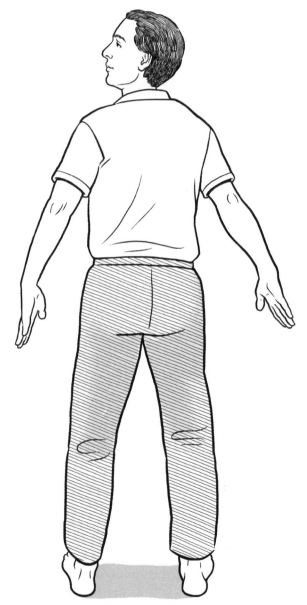

Figure 36: Small Intestine Channel Gesture.

- Filled with the bright red light of the heart your hands find each other palm to palm in front of your root chakra.

- Slowly raise your hands, elbows extended, as if lifting out of a swamp.

- As your arms reach heart height, allow your elbows to bend, bringing your thumbs to your forehead.

- Look skyward and lean gently back in space, "praying to heaven to show the way."

- Finding your truth, come back up standing tall. Gazing straight ahead as you knife your hands forward and down, karate chop edge of your hand leading the way.

- Let your knees bend as you knife forward decisively, hands to either side of your hips, pinky fingers extended behind you.

- Stand tall once more, as you turn your head to look over one shoulder. Breathe out completely.

- As you breathe in look ahead once more, bring your hands back together at the root and repeat the movement up to your forehead and a slight backbend.

- Knife forward once more, exhaling. Bend the knees as the hands go to either side of your hips and stand tall, looking over your other shoulder.

- Repeat this several times, and the last time bring your hands forward to palms press earth and pause there a moment and then move smoothly into the Bladder meridian flow.

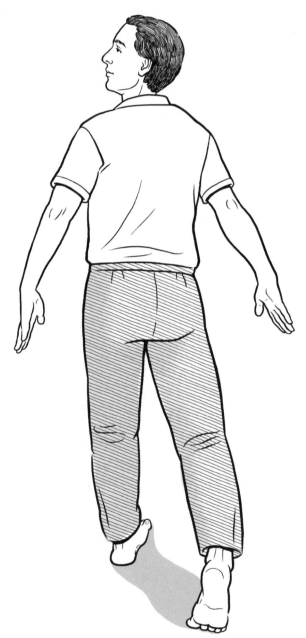

Figure 37: Bladder Channel Gesture.

THE BLADDER CHANNEL GESTURE

To strike a gesture that activates the entire Bladder channel, and illustrates a central feature of its functional range, bring your hands up in front of your body, palms facing the earth. Then swing your hands down along your sides while taking a powerful step forward with one leg, thrusting forward from the midsection of your body. The back heel will come off the ground, articulating the leg all the way down to the pinky toe. To complete the entire gesture, turn your head to look back over the hind foot. As you practice this movement, you will be connecting the entire Bladder channel from Bright Eyes to Extreme Yin. As you do so, say to yourself, "I am driven forward to achieve but I keep an eye on my back!" A strong affirmation that underlines the time honored truth that those who do not learn from the past are doomed to repeat it. Much of the Bladder meridian's functional range can be related to this task.

- With palms pressing earth, shift your weight onto your right foot.

- Step back with your left foot turned inward, in 60/40 stance.

- Shift your weight onto the right front foot once more, sweeping your hands back to either side, and letting your left heel come off the ground.

- Turn your head to look over your right shoulder, twisting as far as you can, as if you could turn and look at your left pinky toe.

- Breathe out completely.

- As you breathe in once more, look front, bring your hands back to palms press earth, and step your right foot back to meet your left.

- Step forward with your left foot, thrusting from your midsection, arms sweeping back to either side again as you shift your weight forward onto the front foot. Your right heel comes off the ground and you turn and look over your left shoulder.

- Step back with the left foot as the hands come forward again to palms press earth. Repeat the affirmation "I drive myself forward, keeping an eye on my back."

- Thrust forward with vigor each time.

- Repeat, alternating sides, many times.

- When complete, sweep arms up and out to the sides, step wide with feet turned out, ready to begin the Kidney gesture.

THE KIDNEY CHANNEL GESTURE

The Kidney channel flows up from the bottoms of the feet to the groin, and from the pubic bone to the clavicle quite near the front centerline of the body. It accesses and governs the deep and personal aspects of libido, procreation, vitality, and ancestral energy that is handed down through the generations. It's position deep in the feet and legs, and moving through the groin and onto the front of the body is auspicious and appropriate. The yoga posture known as Reclining Bound Angle pose is a perfect posture for balancing and activating the Kidney channel. In our standing Meridian Gesture sequence we stay on our feet and perform the following Fountain of Life gesture.

- Take a wide stance, with your feet turned out over your big toes.

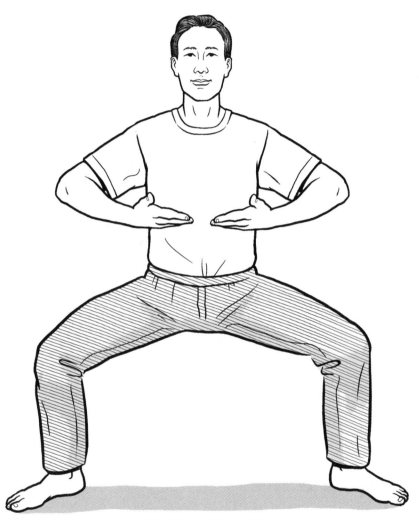

Figure 38: Kidney Channel Gesture.

- In this deep knee bend, sweep your arms down and begin to "gather" the deep yin energies of the earth, as if you were playing in mud or forming clay.

- Continue to shape this clay as you begin to raise the hands up, feeling this earthy energy a deep blue/black, coursing up from the bottom of your foot, through the instep, to the inner ankle, back of the calf, back of the knee, and deep in your thigh from knee to groin.

- As your hands rise to your torso, straighten your spine to an upright posture, keeping a gentle bend in your knees.

- Bring the energy up through your torso, as if filling up from below. Pause at each chakra center and imagine it is being filled up.

- Fill the root, sacrum, solar plexus, heart, throat, third eye, and crown.

- As your hands pass beyond your crown, open them overhead as in the Heart gesture, and deepen your knee bend.

- Feel the red light of heaven descending and joining with the blue/black of earth, forming a royal purple color in your heart.

- Deepen the knee bend as you hold your hands to the heavens. Join the jing of Kidney with the shen in the Heart, unifying yin and yang, earth and heaven.

- Sweep your hands out to the sides and down to the earth to gather once more.

- Repeat three times, and on the last sweep, let the hands rest on your knees and shift weight side to side, building deep strength in the lower extremities.

- As you practice the actions, repeat the words "I feel the vital life force that flows deep within me." With this movement you can positively activate the Kidney channel, filling up your deep center with vital energy.

THE PERICARDIUM CHANNEL GESTURE

Taking the entire meridian length into view, from the breast out through the biceps to the palm of the hand, one can seen the inside circlet of the embracing arms. Here the shared warmth of the heart is demonstrated, a perfect illustration of the meaning and purpose of this meridian in our lives, promoting circulation, shared warmth, and emotional protection. Use the following movements to open the entire channel and energize its function. In the complete sequence, this follows directly after the Kidney gesture.

- Standing up from the deep stance of Kidney, slowly walk your feet together with a toe-heel movement, and bring your palms together in front of your sternum or heart center.

- Pause here a moment and return to oneness. Feel your heartbeat.

- Raise the elbows out to the sides, pressing the hands together more firmly.

- Turn the fingers to face the front and while continuing to keep pressure between the palms, extend the arms out as far as they will go in front of you, keeping them at shoulder height.

- Drop the chest in and back, and feel your shoulder blades stretch and open up, pulling away from the midline of your back.

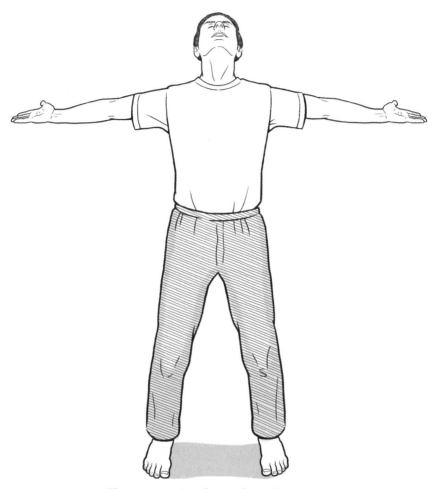

Figure 39: Pericardium Channel Gesture.

- Leading with the fingers, bend the hands back and open them away from one another, slowly but surely opening the arms out to the sides and back in space while keeping them at shoulder height.

- Lead this movement with the middle finger, stretching the palm of the hand as you do so.

- As your arms widen out to your sides, you'll notice the chest naturally opening and expanding forward and a deep breath coming into your chest.

- Continue to move your arms back in space, keeping the hands at shoulder height.

- Stretch back, as if you could touch your middle fingers together behind you.

- Gently lift your gaze heavenward, and hold the stretch for a few breaths, affirming that you open your heart to all the gifts that life has to give you. Let your chest move forward and then your hips, taking yourself into a deep opening stretch.

- Then as you exhale, slowly return your torso to upright, and begin to sweep your hands forward. This leads directly into the Triple Warmer gesture.

THE TRIPLE WARMER CHANNEL GESTURE

To articulate the entire Triple Warmer channel we perform the gesture known as the Bear Hug Twist. It follows neatly after the Pericardium gesture.

- After the wide heart open stretch position of Pericardium, your arms slowly drift forward in a large arc as if you were hugging a large tree.

- Slowly tighten the embrace until you are hugging an imaginary friend.

- Continue to tighten the embrace until you are hugging yourself, your hands wrapped around your shoulders.

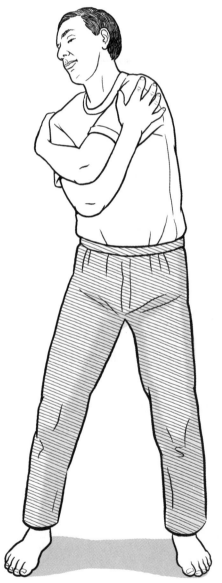

Figure 40: Triple Warmer Channel Gesture.

- As you deepen into this self-embrace, begin to twist gently toward one side, sinking the leading shoulder as you do so. After twisting as far as is comfortable to the side, slowly begin to raise your shoulder, twisting back the other way.

- As you cross midline your leading shoulder will again dip as you move into the twist, and then rise again as you twist back toward centerline.

- Pass centerline once more repeating the dipping twisting, rising, and twisting back the other way, many times.

- Create a smooth figure eight pattern with your movements and begin to luxuriate in the sense of delicious movement, hugging yourself gently and warmly.

- In your mind, or out loud, say to yourself, " I protect myself from all that would harm me." Repeat this several times until you feel a sense of completion.

- Slow the movement down to stillness, facing forward, allowing your hands to slide down the backs of your arms.

THE GALL BLADDER CHANNEL GESTURE

The strong gesture of the Gall Bladder channel is found when you enter the 60/40 stance of kung fu, make fists and hold them in readiness, one forward and one back. Assuming this stance flows naturally out of the previously held Triple Warmer gesture.

- As your hands slide down the backs of your arms from the Triple Warmer gesture, make fists, step forward with left fist and foot into 60/40 Left Forward stance. Left fist holds at the level of your face, right fist back at the level of your hip.

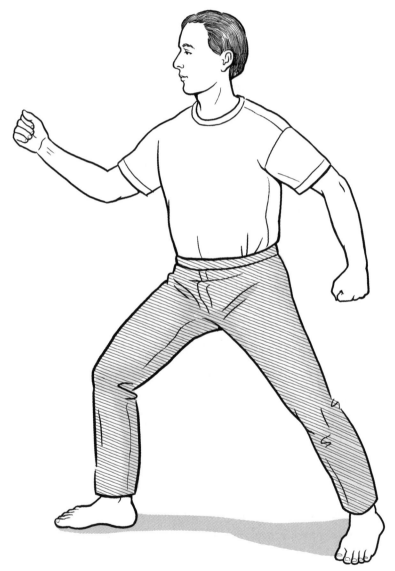

Figure 41: Gall Bladder Channel Gesture.

- Hold the stance firmly and repeat to yourself, "I stand my ground, with strength and integrity." There is a spiritual law that says, "No being may invade another being's territory without permission." You have a right to know and defend your territory from unwanted intrusion.

- Swing the right foot and fist forward, pivoting on the left foot, into 60/40 Right Forward stance.

- Be light on your heels, and launch off the ball mounts of your feet. Pivot on the right foot, as you swing the left fist and foot forward once more into Left Forward stance.

- Launch off the ball mounts as you step back and back again.

- Step forward and forward again.

- Step forward and back repeatedly, launching, landing, and pivoting on the ball mounts of your feet.

- Swing your fists in concert with your feet with each step. Alternately assume the 60/40 Left and Right Forward stance positions with each step.

- Let your breath meet the exertion, exhaling boldly as your moving foot lands.

- Connect to a sense of generating inner power as you make your advance and retreat.

- Surge forward undaunted.

- Retreat and yield with honor.

- Build these skills with poise. Both prove necessary in the many and vast situations of life that call for responsible decision-making.

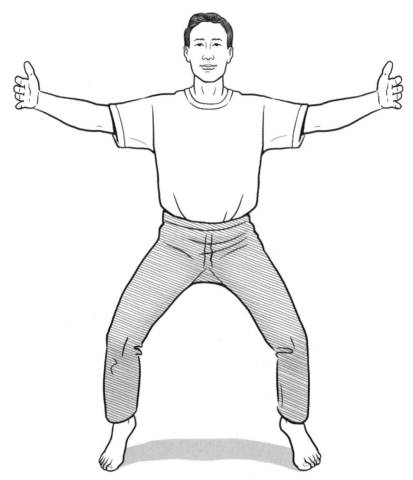

Figure 42: Liver Channel Gesture.

THE LIVER CHANNEL GESTURE

The Liver channel runs a course from the big toe up to the lower ribs. It tracks along the inner calf and thigh, and its position in the legs might best be described by the image of riding on a horse. It can be found all along the surface area of the legs that would be up against the horse's body. When leaving the legs it crosses the area between the hip bone and the pubic bone, and rises up to the lower ribs.

- Coming out of 60/40 Left or Right Forward stance of the Gall Bladder gesture, bring your feet parallel about two shoulder widths apart.

- Gradually un-weight your heels, and rise up on the balls of your feet, balancing on the big toe.

- As you raise up on your feet, lift your arms up and out to the side at chest height, as if you are holding a beach ball twice the size of your torso.

- Stand and hold this position, looking straight ahead.

- With your inner felt sense, follow the Liver channel from the big toe to Liver 3, Excessive Rush. See yourself in the marketplace of life rushing about from task to task.

- Continue up the channel to Liver 10, Leg Five Miles, in the inner thigh, and feel the quality of stamina and endurance building within you.

- Follow the line up through the lymph nodes at the inguinal triangle, cross the abdomen to the eleventh rib, Liver 13, Camphorwood Gate, and feel the metabolism of all your experiences into nourishment and sustenance.

- Bring your attention to Liver 14, Gate of Completion, and feel complete with all your tasks.

- Finally, follow an internal branch of the Liver meridian up to the crown of your head, and stand at the mountaintop with a pure vision for your life.

- Say to yourself: "I envision my life with clarity and purpose."

- Maintain the pose for at least two to eight minutes. Continually repeat the affirmation as you stand in balance and truly allow the feeling of living your life purpose, fulfilling your wildest dream, to course through your body, heartmind, and spirit.

4. Closing Movements—Completing Your Practice Set

After completing the sequence of twelve gestures, we find ourselves in a deeply satisfying ecstatic state of ease and calm produced by our cultivation. We stand in wuji once more, taking a moment to integrate the benefits of the meridian gestures, and we begin a gentle swaying as if we were a supple young willow being wafted by a gentle breeze. This gentle soft movement is natural and deep, organic, and unforced, and leads us softly and sweetly into our closing movements, a time in which we feel deeply merged with the great power of the universe, that which effortlessly keeps the planets circulating around the sun, the earth spinning on its axis, the moon moving through its phases.

Slowly come out of wuji and perform the Infinity Wave and Hands Passing Clouds movements. Doing so will bring your practice into that feeling of a great river flowing to the sea. End with a Radiant Heart Gesture, Pulling Down the Heavens to store the benefits of your practice deep in the marrow of your bones. Offer a deep bow in gratitude for the practice and your connection to all that is.

After the full practice of Meridian Gesture Qigong, you now arrive at these elegant completion gestures where you take the qi that you have cultivated and integrate the benefits of the practice deep into the core of your being. To this end, the classical practices of Infinity Wave, Hands Passing Clouds, Polishing the Stone, and Radiant Heart Gesture–Pulling Down the Heavens are perfectly suited.

Follow along with the instructions below, and let these movements take you deep into union with all that is, dissolving into the fields of life of which you are an integral part.

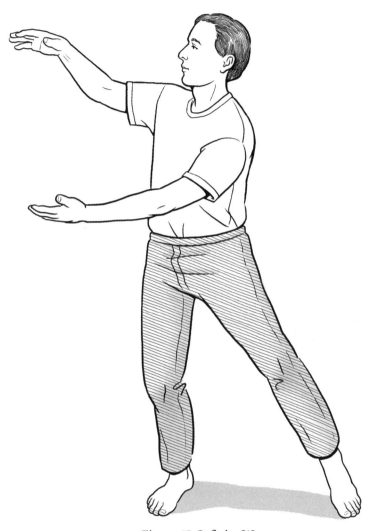

Figure 43: Infinity Wave.

Infinity Wave

- Standing in wuji, allow your hands to float up in front of your torso, about the height of the solar plexus.

- Face the right palm up and the left palm down.

- Turn your body to the right, sweeping your hands right as well.

- At the extremity of your turn, turn your palms over and begin to sweep back to the left.

- Reach the extremity toward the left and turn the palms over once more, turning again to the right.

- Continue this side to side gesture, turning the palms over and gliding smoothly through the movements, tracing a figure eight, Infinity Wave in the air.

Hands Passing Clouds: Looking Near, Looking Far

- Coming out of Infinity Wave as you are turning toward the left, raise the left hand to the level of your eyes, palm facing you, and stare into the center of your palm. Your right hand will face the earth.

- When you reach the extremity of your turn to the left, slowly lower the left hand and gaze off into the distance as your right hand rises to the level of your eyes.

- Face the right palm toward your face and gaze into the center of the right palm as you turn back to the right.

- At the extremity of the turn to the right, the right hand drops and you gaze into the distance as the left hand rises to face you at eye level.

- Gaze once more into the palm as you turn.

- Between you and your palm is all you. Beyond the back of your palm lie the ten thousand things.

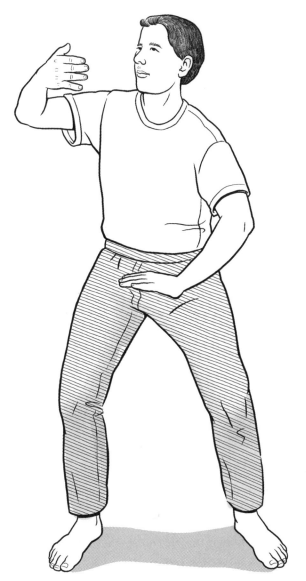

Figure 44: Hand Passing Clouds.

POLISHING THE STONE: THE ART OF BALANCE AND CULTIVATING SMOOTH QI FLOW

- Attain a classic 60/40 stance.

- Palms press earth—bring the palms forward, facing the ground, in front of hips at the height of t'an t'ien.

- Shift the weight forward onto the front foot.

- Smoothly turn the hips 45 degrees toward the back foot while sweeping the hands sideways as if polishing the surface of a marble counter top. Bring the weight back to the back foot in one smooth motion as the hands move back to the waist.

- Turn the hips to square with front foot once more, shift weight to front foot, and sweep hands forward and around to the side. Once more, shift the weight back to the back foot, returning the hands to the waist.

- Repeat many times.

- Switch sides. Bring front foot back, back foot front, sweep to the second side.

RADIANT HEART GESTURE: DANCING HEAVEN TO EARTH

- Opening your awareness to the infinite interplay of yin and yang—once more connect to your body's toroidal magnetic field.

  - Call to mind the shape of an apple or orange, activate your awareness of the luminous sphere of light that emanates from your center and surrounds your entire body.

- Yang: Pulling Down the Heavens—Gathering of Light— yang energy moves down through the core, dispersing down into the earth.

- Breathing in, sweep your arms down and out to sides gathering the soil, water, wind. Smoothly sweep your hands up toward the sky and gather the light of the sun, moon, and stars. Slowly breathe out, as you press your hands down through the midline of the body.
- Repeat Pulling Down the Heavens three times.
- On the third time, bring your hands together at your heart center and bow in gratitude toward yourself for bringing yourself through your practice. Acknowledge yourself for your practice and take the benefits deep into your soul.

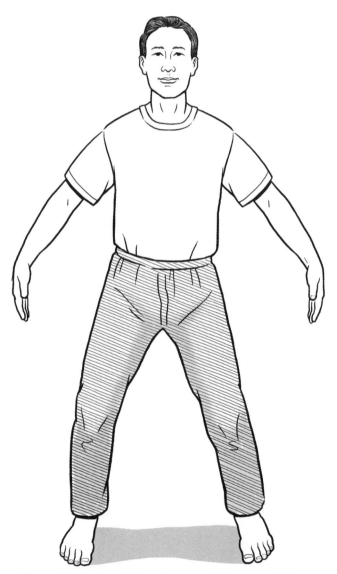

Figure 45: Radiant Heart Gesture: Gathering of Light—
Pulling Down the Heavens 1.

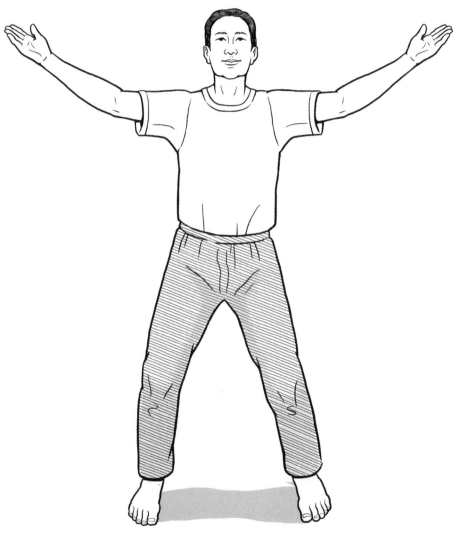

Figure 46: Radiant Heart Gesture: Gathering of Light—
Pulling Down the Heavens 2.

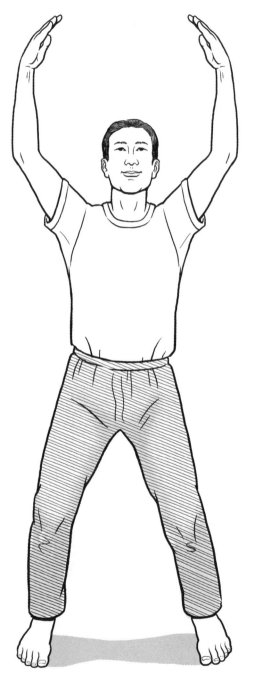

Figure 47: Radiant Heart Gesture: Fountain of Life 1.

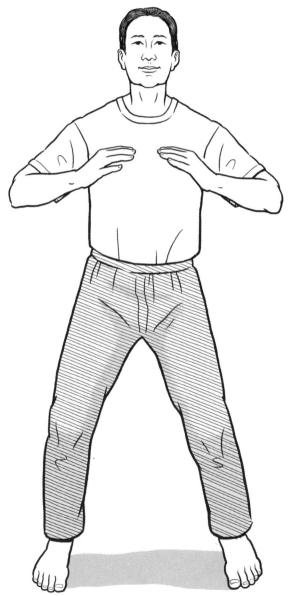

Figure 48: Radiant Heart Gesture: Fountain of Life 2.

Conclusion

Revisiting the Pathways of Qi

In all this detailed study of the twelve regular channels, we Westerners can easily get caught up in our intellect and our lists. We love our lists! I'm certain I'm guilty of this myself. And I would be remiss to end this book filled with all its marvelously detailed lists without steering these hungry intellects back to the title of the work. The theme that carries this whole work through is not the many pathways of qi but rather the one pathway of qi.

And as I was taught in my practice over the years, I extend here in *Pathways of Qi* the cautionary teaching, "Don't get caught up in the twelve, see them only as aspects of the one!" In deeply internalizing all these aspects you come back to an important question when approaching the whole. "What shows up missing?" If you truly know the whole, then the one piece that has been neglected will be obvious in its absence.

There is one energy that flows throughout the body, heartmind, and spirit, and it is only with this understanding firmly in place that we can deeply appreciate the many aspects of being. Where we point the camera, we take a picture. The trick is to see the whole as it expresses itself in each aspect. Like the story of the five blind men who each touch a different part of the elephant, there are many impressions that come from each distinct part. Our work is to always see each part in the context of the whole.

It is an unfortunate part of Western culture that so many people have lost sight of the whole. In Western medicine for instance are drugs that treat the liver but damage the kidneys or treat the heart but damage the lungs... and so forth. Always honing in on one part, we may benefit that part to a certain extent, but if the whole is not taken into account serious imbalance can follow.

Ultimately, the balance of the whole must always be of utmost consideration. One way of saying this for the practitioner of the Eastern medical approach is "We don't treat disease. We support balance. As balance is restored, we watch the disease go away."

Through compassionate awareness of the whole, we can learn to use the various expressions that arise from our study of each aspect of our one meridian flow. The twelve organ networks each express themselves in constitution, character, and temperament, excess and deficient patterns, the daily cycle of energy flow, and the movement of life energy throughout the body's interconnected energetic systems. And it is through embracing the interconnection that we can create the life we want. A life of vibrancy, balance, and health is within reach for each of us. Knowing the one meridian flow and its many faces expressing through organ networks and their characteristic manifestations provides us with a powerful tool to discern where we are on the path of life.

Balance is an art and a science. Use the lists but don't get caught up in them. See them as a part of a greater whole. Notice when one aspect has become strong or dominant, and what aspect has become weak through neglect. Build up your abilities slowly and consistently, touch on every part of the wheel. Check every spoke, and make sure the hub is sound. In this way the wheel of life will continue spinning perfectly. Use your breath and consciousness, develop your awareness, and flow forward with ease and grace through all of life's many blessings. Allow the pathway of qi to guide you forward with grace.

Granted, this book has not spoken in great detail about the hub; rather it has focused on awakening your awareness and understanding of the wheel's many spokes. The art is now to see how they are all interconnected. When approaching the actual central force binding them all together, you enter the realm of the study of qi itself, the very life force that animates and governs all the functions of the body, heartmind, and spirit. It is my hope that you will carry this consciousness forward into your work. And so I conclude this work with the final instruction: Keep striving toward the awareness of the whole. Do not lose sight of the forest for the trees, but let your awareness of one tree inform you of the forest's might and health with reverence and love.

To this end, the arts of qigong, shiatsu, breath, and meditation are key. After all your study, quiet your mind, connect to your spirit with love, and truly appreciate the tremendous flow of life. It is said that the mind guides the qi, but what guides the mind? The classics answer resolutely: "Spirit guides the mind." Learn to let spirit guide you, and the qi energy of your life will flow freely and clearly through all aspects of your being.

It seems deeply appropriate that at the end of all this study, I bring you to a starting point—love. With love of life, love of energy, love of learning, and love of the delicate and intricate expressions of qi, you will come to awaken within, having a sense of true and deep loving connection to all that is. In this way, you will come to know for yourself in your true heart the pathways of qi.

Recommended Resources

Invitation to Further Study

If this work has intrigued you, I urge you to study further. I am building a library of works around the HeartMind Bodywork philosophy and approach to life and healing. I also operate ongoing training programs worldwide to bring this message directly to those in need. We are looking for committed individuals who sense a calling here to develop their skills and abilities in this way of being. Please contact my institute through the following web pages for more information on how you may take your study and practice further.

www.matthewsweigart.com

www.heartmindbodywork.com

Full Color Meridian Gestures and Functions Chart

The full-color wall chart on this website brings you a visual representation of the twelve regular channels in the daily cycle of meridian energy flow rendered in a beautiful lotus wheel. Included are major points, six divisions, temperament traits, five element wheel, and Master Masunaga's front and back diagnostic areas.

www.matthewsweigart.com/products-page/charts/heartmind
 -shiatsu-chart/

Meridian Tapping Video Course

This three-and-a-half-hour online video course guides you through a complete sequence of meridian tapping of the twelve regular channels in seven jam-packed half-hour lessons.

www.matthewsweigart.com/products-page/dvds/meridian-tapping/

Meridian Gesture Qigong Video Course

This twelve-hour online video course brings you a thorough training in the Meridian Gesture Qigong method with full guidance in warm-ups, classical movements, and meridian gestures and functions.

www.matthewsweigart.com/products-page/dvds/meridians
 -12-qigong-teacher-training-level-1-dvd-set/

Harmonizing Heaven and Earth DVD

This full length DVD brings you sixty-five minutes of beautiful footage covering the basic qi cultivation methods, as well as a full overview of the HeartMind Bodywork Shiatsu Therapy practice. Beginning, Intermediate, Advanced, and Advanced Flying techniques are demonstrated to give you a full experience of the scope of HeartMind Shiatsu Asian Bodywork Therapy.

www.matthewsweigart.com/products-page/dvds/harmonizing
 -heaven-and-earth-dvd/

Appendix

Acupoint Name Reference Guide

Following are English translations of the names of all the acupoints on the twelve regular channels as used in the HeartMind Shiatsu school of Asian Bodywork Therapy. Correlate these names with the images presented in chapters 2 through 7 in order to develop a more clear picture of the meridian line functions and specific point qualities.

The nomenclature of acupuncture has been developed over thousands of years. I include here a list of translations from the Chinese drawn from a variety of trusted sources and my own clinical applications. The names are true to the original Chinese characters but as with all such translations are subject to great interpretation. In the bibliography, I have listed various sources both on- and offline where you can take your study of point nomenclature deeper if that is your interest. To me, the names are windows into a deep awareness and appreciation for the body's rich, complex, and beautiful functionality.

The names often evoke and describe the point's clinical usage. There are many sources and various translations of the points' names that have appeared in various schools over many years. In addition, many of the points are known to have multiple names. There is an art to the science of the point names, and just reading through the lists can give you a sense for the range and depth of meaning of this powerful system.

By calling to mind the point names as you practice qigong, meditation, or touch therapy you can activate the energy of the point for greater effectiveness. An acupuncturist may use needles, an acupressurist their fingers and thumbs, a shiatsu therapist palms and elbows, knees and feet, as well as thumbs. In all cases, as is true of qigong, we need to use our mind to guide the qi to and through the points and ultimately our spirit to guide the mind. Deep in the work is the understanding that where the mind goes, qi flows.

As you study these point names and correlate them to the place on the body where they are found, bring your mind and imagination to bear upon the discovery of the usefulness of the point. In this way, you exponentially enhance the effectiveness and scope of your self-discovery and healing practice.

Lung—Hand Tai Yin

1. Central Treasury

2. Cloud Gate

3. Palace of Heaven

4. Reaching White

5. Cubit Marsh (In the Groove)

6. Maximum Opening

7. Broken Sequence

8. Channel Gutter

9. Great Abyss

10. Fish Belly

11. Little Merchant

Large Intestine—Hand Yang Ming

1. Yang Merchant

2. Second Space

3. Third Space

4. Meeting Valley

5. Yang Stream (Snuffbox)

6. Veering Passage

7. Warm Flow

8. Lower Angle

9. Upper Angle

10. Arm Three Miles

11. Pool at the Bend

12. Elbow Crevice

13. Arm Five Miles

14. Upper Arm

15. Shoulder Bone

16. Great Bone

17. Heaven's Tripod

18. Support Prominence

19. Mouth Crevice

20. Welcome Fragrance

Stomach—Foot Yang Ming

1. Tear Receptacle
2. Four Whites
3. Great Crevice
4. Earth Granary
5. Great Welcome
6. Jaw Bone
7. Below the Joint
8. Head Bound
9. Welcome Human
10. Water Prominence
11. Abode of Qi
12. Empty Basin
13. Qi Door
14. Storehouse
15. Room Divider
16. Breast Window
17. Breast Center
18. Breast Root
19. Not Contained
20. Supporting Fitness
21. Beam Gate
22. Pass Gate
23. Supreme Unity
24. Slippery Flesh Gate
25. Celestial Pivot

26. Outer Mound

27. The Great

28. Water Passage

29. Return

30. Qi Thoroughfare

31. Thigh Gate

32. Crouching Rabbit

33. Yin Market

34. Ridge Mound

35. Calf's Nose

36. Leg Three Miles

37. Upper Great Hall

38. Ribbon Passage Way

39. Lower Great Hall

40. Bountiful Bulge

41. Stream Divide

42. Rushing Yang

43. Sunken Valley

44. Inner Courtyard

45. Severe Mouth

Spleen—Foot Tai Yin

1. Hidden White

2. Great Metropolis

3. Supreme White

4. Grandfather Grandson (Yellow Emperor)

5. Trade Winds Mound

6. Three Yin Meeting

7. Granary Hole

8. Earth's Crux

9. Yin Mound Spring

10. Sea of Blood

11. Winnower's Gate

12. Rushing Gate

13. Abode of the Yin Organs

14. Abdomen Knot

15. Great Horizontal

16. Abdomen Sorrow

17. Food Cavity

18. Heavenly Stream

19. Chest Village

20. Encircling Glory

21. Great Embracement

Heart—Hand Shao Yin

1. Highest Spring

2. Cyan Spirit

3. Lesser Sea

4. Spirit Path

5. Penetrating the Interior

6. Yin Cleft

7. Spirit Gate

8. Lesser Palace

9. Lesser Rushing

Small Intestine—Hand Tai Yang

1. Lesser Marsh

2. Front Valley

3. Back Stream

4. Wrist Bone

5. Yang Valley

6. Support the Aged

7. Upright Branch

8. Small Sea

9. Correct Shoulder

10. Upper Arm Transport

11. Heavenly Gathering

12. Grasping the Wind

13. Crooked Wall

14. Outer Shoulder Transport

15. Middle Shoulder Transport

16. Heavenly Window

17. Divine Appearance

18. Cheek Bone Hole

19. Palace of Hearing

Bladder—Foot Tai Yang

1. Bright Eyes

2. Silk Bamboo Bone

3. Eyebrows' Pouring

4. Crooked Curve

5. Fifth Palace

6. Receiving Light

7. Heavenly Connection

8. Declining Connection

9. Jade Pillow

10. Celestial Pillar

11. Great Shuttle

12. Wind Gate

13. Lung Transporter

14. Pericardium Transporter

15. Heart Transporter

16. Governor Transporter

17. Diaphragm Transporter

18. Liver Transporter

19. Gall Bladder Transporter

20. Spleen Transporter

21. Stomach Transporter

22. Triple Warmer Transporter

23. Kidney Transporter (Vitality Gate)

24. Sea of Qi Transporter

25. Large Intestine Transporter

26. Origin Gate Transporter

27. Small Intestine Transporter

28. Bladder Transporter

29. Mid Spine Transporter

30. White Ring Transporter

31. Upper Crevice

32. Second Crevice

33. Middle Crevice

34. Lower Crevice

35. Meeting of Yang

36. Brings Relief

37. Gate of Abundance

38. Floating Cleft

39. Outside the Crook

40. Middle of the Crook

41. Attached Branch

42. Door of the Corporeal Soul

43. Vital Region Transporter

44. Hall of the Spirit

45. Yi Xi

46. Diaphragm Gate

47. Gate of the Ethereal Soul

48. Yang's Key Link

49. Abode of Consciousness

50. Stomach Granary

51. Vitals Gate

52. Residence of the Will

53. Bladder's Vitals

54. Order's Limit

55. Confluence of Yang

56. Support the Sinews

57. In the Mountains

58. Flying Yang

59. Instep Yang

60. Kunlun Mountains

61. Servant's Respect

62. Extending Vessel

63. Golden Gate

64. Capital Bone

65. Restraining Bone

66. Foot Connecting Valley

67. Extreme Yin

Kidney—Foot Shao Yin

1. Bubbling Spring

2. Blazing Valley

3. Supreme Stream

4. Great Bell

5. Water Spring

6. Shining Sea

7. Returning Current

8. Exchange Belief

9. Guest House

10. Yin Valley

11. Pubic Bone

12. Great Luminance

13. Qi Cave

14. Fourfold Fullness

15. Middle Flow

16. Vitals Transporter

17. Trade Winds Bend

18. Stone Pass

19. Yin Metropolis

20. Abdomen Connecting Valley

21. Mysterious Gate

22. Walking Corridor

23. Spirit Seal

24. Spirit Ruin

25. Spirit Storehouse

26. Comfortable Chest

27. Transporter (Elegant) Mansion

Pericardium—Hand Jue Yin

1. Heaven's Pond

2. Heavenly Spring

3. Marsh at the Crook

4. Xi-Cleft Gate

5. Intermediate Messenger

6. Inner Frontier Gate

7. Great Mound

8. Palace of Toil

9. Central Rushing

Triple Warmer—Hand Shao Yang

1. Rushing Pass

2. Fluid Gate

3. Central Islet

4. Yang Pool

5. Outer Frontier Gate

6. Branch Ditch

7. Ancestral Meeting

8. Three Yang Meeting

9. Four Rivers

10. Heavenly Will

11. Clear Cold Abyss

12. Dispersing River

13. Upper Arm Meeting

14. Shoulder Crevice

15. Heavenly Crevice

16. Window of Heaven

17. Wind Screen

18. Spasm Vessel

19. Skull's Rest

20. Minute Angle

21. Ear Gate

22. Ear Harmony Crevice

23. Silk Bamboo Hollow

Gall Bladder—Foot Shao Yang

1. Seeing the World

2. Meeting of Hearing

3. Above the Joint

4. Jaw Serenity

5. Wild Skull

6. Wild Tuft

7. Crook of the Temple

8. Leading Valley

9. Heavenly Rushing

10. Many Voices

11. Inner Listening

12. Getting into Action

13. Root of the Spirit

14. Yang White (Third Eye Opening)

15. Head Overlooking Tears

16. Window of the Eyes (See the Face of God)

17. Upright Nourishment (God Sees You)

18. Supporting Spirit

19. Brain Hollow

20. Pond of Wind

21. Well in the Shoulder

22. Armpit Abyss

23. Flank Sinews

24. Sun and Moon

25. Capital Gate

26. Girdling Vessel

27. Five Pivots

28. Linking Path

29. Stationary Crevice

30. Jumping Pivot

31. Market of Wind

32. Middle Ditch

33. Knee Yang Gate

34. Yang Mound Spring

35. Yang Intersection

36. Outer Hill

37. Bright Light

38. Yang Assistance

39. Suspended Bell

40. Mound of Ruins

41. Foot Overlooking Tears

42. Earth Five Meetings

43. Clamped Stream

44. Foot Yin Portal

Liver—Foot Jue Yin

1. Great Pile

2. Between Columns

3. Great Rushing

4. Middle Seal

5. Shell Groove

6. Middle Capital

7. Knee Pass

8. Spring at the Bend

9. Yin Envelope

10. Leg Five Miles

11. Yin Screen

12. Rapid Pulse

13. Camphorwood Gate

14. Gate of the Cycle

Major Acupoint Quick Reference Names and Applications

Here is a compendium of the major points and a shorthand reference to how they might be used in treatment. There are some alternate names in this list. Do not be thrown by that. There are many traditions and lineages that have worked with these points, and different names can give you additional information on how they might be used.

Lung

1 Center of Gathering	Respiratory Health
2 Cloud Gate	Moistening
5 In the Groove	Holding on Too Tightly
9 Great Abyss	Letting Go
11 Little Merchant	Energy Exchange

Large Intestine

1 Yang Merchant	Material Exchange
4 Joining Valleys	Elimination, Well-Being
10 Arm Three Miles	Keeping your Grip
15 Corner of the Shoulder	Shoulder Pain
20 Welcome Fragrance	Sinus Congestion

Stomach

8 Head Band	Mental Faculties
9 Man's Prognosis	General Health
25 Celestial Pivot	Intestinal Health
30 Qi Thoroughfare	Energy to Lower Extremities
36 Leg Three Miles	Endurance, Well-Being
40 Bountiful Bulge	Clearing Excesses
41 Shoelace	Ankle Strength

Spleen

4 Yellow Emperor	Digestive Health
6 Three Yin Meeting	Menstrual Cycle
9 Yin Mound Spring	Bodily Dampness
10 Sea of Blood	Vital Energy
11 Winnower's Gate	Separating Pure from Impure
20 Great Embracement	Harmonizing Energy

Heart

1 Highest Spring	Relieving Heart Congestion
2 Cyan Spirit	Opening Circulation
3 Lesser Sea	Calming Nerves
7 Gate of God	Soothing Spirit
9 Lesser Surge	Steady the Heart

Small Intestine

4 Wrist Bone	Balance the Opposites
6 Curing the Aged	Steady the Hand
11 Center of Heaven	Clear the Mind
12 Grasping the Wind	Common Cold
19 Palace of Hearing	Opening the Ears

Bladder

1 Bright Eyes	Open and Close the Eyes
10 Pillar of Heaven	Occipital Headache
13 Lung associated	Breathing
14 Pericardium associated	Circulation
15 Heart associated	Communication
18 Liver associated	Addictions
19 Gall Bladder associated	Responsibility
20 Spleen associated	Digestion
21 Stomach associated	Appetite
22 Triple Warmer associated	Immune System
23 Kidney associated	Vitality
25 Large Intestine associated	Elimination
27 Small Intestine associated	Assimilation
28 Bladder associated	Drive
57 In the Mountains	Frustration, Fatigue
67 Extreme Yin	Labor Pains

Kidney

1 Gushing Spring	Revitalize
3 Great Ravine	Trauma
10 Yin Valley	Constitutional Issues
13 Infant's Door	Fertility

21 Dark Gate | Inner Resources
27 Elegant Mansion | Vital Reserves

Pericardium

1 Heaven's Pond | Lactation
3 Marsh at the Bend | "Tennis" Elbow
6 Inner Gate | Self-Love
8 Palace of Anxiety | Easing Nerves
9 Central Nexus | Developing Strategy

Triple Warmer

5 Outer Gate | Love of Others
10 Heaven's Well | Cooling Tempers
15 Heaven's Bone | Burdens
23 Silk Bamboo Hollow | Heat Strain Headache

Gall Bladder

20 Pond of Wind | Whirlwind Headache
21 Well in the Shoulder | Responsibility
24 Sun and Moon | Gall Bladder Illness
25 Capital Gate | Kidney Illness
30 Jumping Pivot | Hip Challenges, Sciatica
31 Market of Wind | Over-Responsibility
34 Yang Mound Spring | Sinews, Muscles
41 Foot Overlooking Tears | Releasing Excess Holding

Liver

3 Excessive Rush | Slowing Down
4 Middle Seal | Muscle Relaxer
10 Leg Five Miles | Stamina
13 Camphorwood Gate | Digestive Issues
14 Gate of the Cycle | Completion

Bibliography of Sources

Following is a general bibliography of the major influences on this book and my life's work in the healing arts. I am deeply grateful to have been exposed to this body of knowledge in my life. It is my earnest endeavor in this work to create a complete sense of the meridian system and its workings, though it would be presumptuous to suggest that my slender volume could possibly capture the full range and power of this intricate and beautiful system. I encourage the curious reader to study more, read more, practice more, and to bring the meridian knowledge alive in their own being. The following list is a good place to start.

Beinfield, Harriet, and Efrem Korngold, *Between Heaven and Earth: A Guide to Chinese Medicine.* New York: Ballantine Books, 1991.

These expert clinicians offer us beautiful five element interpretations of personality in their landmark text.

Connelley, Dianne M. *All Sickness Is Homesickness.* Columbia, MD: Wisdom Well Press, 1993.

This deeply poetic work explores the mysteries and practices of the four examinations offering deep insight and practical guidance on the path of reading the body, heartmind, and spirit energy.

Dürckheim, Kalfried Graf. *Hara: The Vital Center of Man.* London: George Allen & Unwin, 1962.

This is a classic rendering of the Japanese self-cultivation practices and methods for achieving personal mastery.

Hammer, Leon. *Dragon Rises, Red Bird Flies.* Seattle: Eastland Press, 2005.

Many intricate and sophisticated correlations between Chinese medicine and Western psychology are eloquently drawn out in this powerful exposition.

Jahnke, Roger. *The Healing Promise of Qi: Creating Extraordinary Wellness Through Qigong and Tai Chi.* New York: McGraw-Hill, 2002.

Elucidates the Chinese Medical system and the practices of personal cultivation of life energy.

Jarrett, Lonny. *Nourishing Destiny: The Inner Tradition of Chinese Medicine.* Richmond, MA: Spirit Path Press, 2009.

This engaging work is a deeply inspiring exploration of the five elements, meridians, and points of Chinese medicine.

Kaptchuk, Ted J. *The Web That Has No Weaver: Understanding Chinese Medicine.* New York: Contemporary Books, 2000.

An excellent volume that clearly states many of the main ideas of the Chinese medical perspective.

Mails, Thomas E. *Fools Crow: Wisdom and Power.* San Francisco: Council Oak Books, 1991.

A profound work describing the life and practices of the master Lakota shaman and healer Fools Crow.

Masunaga, Shizuto, and Wataru Ohashi. *Zen Shiatsu: How to Harmonize Yin and Yang for Better Health.* New York: Japan Publications, 1974.

Offers a powerful introduction to the psychological interpretations of meridian energies.

Requena, Yves. *Character and Health: The Relationship of Acupuncture and Psychology.* Brookline, MA: Paradigm Publications, 1989.

This landmark work interweaves the understanding of the six divisions of yin and yang and Western pathology into the study of constitution and temperament.

Yuen, Jeffrey. *The Eight Extraordinary Vessels.* Watertown, MA: New England School of Acupuncture, Continuing Education Department, 2005.

Jeffrey Yuen's masterful contributions to the field of energetics, particularly in his teachings of classical Chinese medicine, the three levels of health, and the eight extraordinary vessels.

Glossary

Channel—a term that is used to name the qi flow pathways, and capture the characteristic aspect of a vessel that carries a substance from one place to another. The image of a water channel, or a TV channel are both useful in using this term to describe the energy flows in the human body.

Inferior—an anatomical term that refers to a place on the body below, beneath, or closer to the earth than the point or anatomical landmark it is being compared to.

Jing—the most dense material aspect of the essence of spirit as it manifests in the tissues of the body.

Lateral—referring to the side aspects of the body.

Medial—referring to the aspects of the body that are toward the midline of the body.

Meridian—"an imaginary line on the surface of the body," which in this context was a misused term used by European mariners upon first learning of the acupuncture meridian lines of Chinese medicine

Pathway—a trajectory of the qi flow as it expresses itself along the surface of the body.

Qi—the "stuff" of the universe, the universal life energy force, a force so vast and varied that no simple definition could ever possibly convey its deep meaning.

Qigong—Literally "qi cultivation" this term refers to any conscious exercise that is used to raise the awareness and work with the flow of qi energy in the body, heartmind, and spirit.

Shen—The most ethereal, illusive, and ephemeral aspect of the essence of spirit.

Superior—An anatomical term that refers to a place on the body above or closer to the sky than the point or anatomical landmark it is being compared to.

Yin and Yang—Terms used to ascribe the two relative, equal, complementary, relative, and polar opposite forces of nature and the cosmos.

Yin—The earthly, physical, dark aspects of the universe.

Yang—The heavenly, ethereal, light aspects of the universe.

Zang/Fu—The Chinese term used to identify the organ networks of the body, of which the meridian channels are the energetic expression running through the cutaneous regions of the body, and the actual physical organs and their functions are the internal energetic expression. Zang refers to the yin organ networks or viscera, and fu to the yang organ networks or bowels.